FOOD: Is for Life!

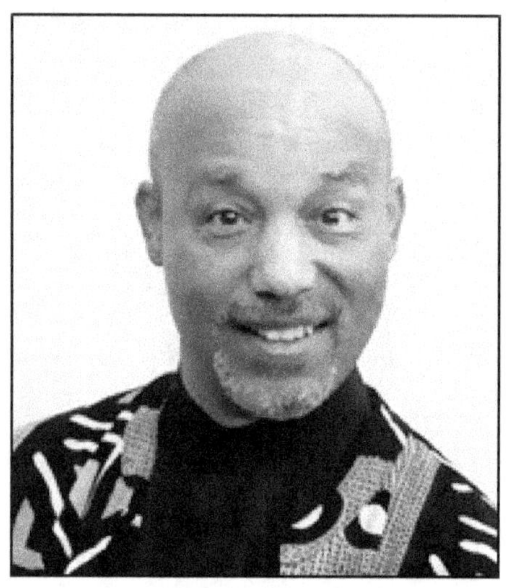

This book is authored by Keidi Awadu.
Copyright 1996 / 2020 update, and published by the Conscious Rasta Press for Black Star Media Global,
Las Vegas, Nevada USA
All rights are reserved under United States copyright law.

Contents

Chapter 1 – Food for Life

Food is Nature's Perfect Medicine

In recent decades, people are increasingly learning to use nutrition to prevent or reverse chronic diseases, mental illness, and reproductive disorders.

Among the most exciting and motivating trends within upwardly mobile circles is the increase in education about the "Western diet" and how it has severely impacted its adherents' health. This information is gushing forth, flowing out from books, magazines, videotapes, and various alternative health forums.

Comedian/activist Dick Gregory, considered a wonderful resource on health, politics, and education, frequently reminds us that "Information is knowledge and knowledge is power."

An extraordinary level of enthusiasm is being generated throughout different strata of society, young and old, rich and poor, for information on nutritional roads to prevent or reverse lifestyle patterns that result in poor health.

There are three particular areas of concern where proper eating has shown to provide impressive health results. They are 1) chronic diseases, 2) mental well-being, and 3) reproductive health. An accumulation of evidence attests that we can eat our way toward longevity, clarity of thought, and vitality.

Whom among us would not wish upon ourselves the blessings of great health, intellectual prowess, and powerful sexual energy? Yet realistic assessment indicates that this will not be accomplished merely by hoping, praying, or clicking our heels while chanting. The path toward nutritional excellence requires alertness on the part of the student. There are countless diversions by charlatans with undisclosed financial motivations. Monopolistic corporations are increasingly underhanded in their spread of mind control through the media to convince us that their product alone will fulfill our dreams of strength, alertness, and sexuality. As the West has been acculturated toward instant gratification and the quick fix, much of the public would prefer to pop a pill, drink a potion or smear on some cream that will rapidly deliver the essential desire. Yet, through correct analysis, we become aware that such promises are usually unfulfilled.

The nutritional road to long-term health and wellness is not a tortured path. Still, it does require a degree of concentration, diligence, consistency, and zeal that result from a lifelong commitment. I hope, through this publication, to assist the reader along that wonderful path. The journey to wholeness requires one not to race along at breakneck speed, but to take firm steps, one accomplishment after another until we have built up sufficient momentum to be able to maintain a steady pace. Among the first realizations to occur to us is that achieving optimal health is an enjoyable, satisfying task.

Epidemic Rates of "Modern Diseases"

Escherichia coli (also known as E. coli), "flesh-eating bacteria," AIDS, Ebola, hantavirus, "mad cow disease," antibiotic-resistant bugs – we are increasingly bombarded with terrifying propaganda in the media with threats of plagues from these exotic "new" diseases which might one day rampage uncontrollably within certain population groups.

Yet, the reality is slightly more mundane. Though the mind controllers and social engineers would leave us hysterical over the prospect of plague epidemics, the fact is that other, less compelling, diseases are working their deadly toll on the public. When we analyze mortality statistics related to cancer, heart, kidney, liver and thyroid disease, hypertension, diabetes, stroke, obesity, and other common ailments – this is where widespread concern should be focused.

Is it possible that the media hasn't given focus to the more mundane disease killers because such disorders are largely either preventable or manageable through proper diet and nutrition? Still, such lifestyle modifications are contrary to the interests of corporate sponsors of major media outlets?

By now, we should all be aware of the healthy benefits of fresh fruits and vegetables, plenty of pure water, non-meat diets, avoidance of toxins, pesticides, petrochemicals, etc. Yet, when was the last time one saw a commercial for broccoli, yams, green beans, or spinach? We are continuously bombarded, from infancy, with advertisements for alcoholic beverages, tobacco, candy, pastry, sodas, quick fixes, greasy fast food, and other consumable products.

Further, the propagandists would have us believe that dairy products, candy bars, hyper-sweetened drinks, and pork ("the other white meat") are in actuality either proper eating or conducive to more energy and vitality.

Could there be a demonstrable link between such poor dietary habits and the chronic diseases which claim the greatest numbers of deaths? What are these common disease killers?

Four Leading Disease Killers in the U.S.

Heart Disease

Heart disease generally falls into two categories, congenital (developed at birth) and acquired. As we are dealing specifically with the dietary links to this, the major killer in the industrialized countries, we will concern ourselves with acquired heart disease.

The majority of heart disease is related to constriction of the blood vessels, called coronary heart disease, which results in the muscle being overworked and clogging of the organ itself, which leads in a vast majority of cases to congestive heart failure.

The sad fact is that such dietary influences as excess cholesterol consumption, smoking, alcohol, obesity, and the sedentary lifestyle – all controllable factors –have been linked to the fairly recent outbreak of heart disease (coronary heart disease only became epidemic as late as the 1960s). It should be noted that not all countries have a high rate of heart disease that seems to plague the industrialized nations disproportionately. Also noted is the relationship between other chronic diseases such as hypertension and diabetes to increased heart disease risk.

Though medical science has claimed remarkable strides in managing heart disease, or in the absence of prevention to be able to replace the "broken" heart with a fresh one, the mainstream medical establishment has been somewhat negligent in policing those environmental influences which have largely contributed to the plague that heart disease has become.

Rather than relying upon pacemakers, defibrillation devices, bypass operations, nitroglycerin pills, transplants, and other high-tech solutions, it would perhaps be best to instill those habits early in life that environmental influences which promote heart disease later in life can be avoided.

Cancer

Environmental influences, including diet, smoking, alcoholic beverages, occupation, chemical exposure, and geographic location, account for over 60 percent of all cancers. The International Agency for Research on Cancer has "identified 60 environmental agents that can cause cancer," including chemicals, groups of related chemicals, chemical mixtures, radiation, drugs, and occupational exposures. Nutrition is believed to affect at least 35% of cancers directly. Cancer has risen for all ages, and 70% of cancers are unrelated to smoking.

White male Baby Boomers suffer three times the cancer rate of their grandfathers, and white women of the same generation are 30% more likely to develop cancers unrelated to smoking than their grandmothers. Cancer is the leading killer of children in the U.S.

Colorectal cancer is the nation's leading cancer killer. An estimated 134,500 Americans develop the disease each year. The link between colorectal cancer and diet is almost absolute. Indicators such as frequent constipation and severe hemorrhoids are hints that a person is en route to developing the disease. The low amount of fiber in the standard Yankee diet is the single greatest risk factor for colorectal cancer. It should be noted that African-Americans consume on average about 15 to 20% of the fiber eaten by their African counterparts. Colorectal cancer is rare in Central East Africa, where fiber consumption is in excess of 70 grams each day compared to a mere 12 to 15 grams in the U.S.

Over 44,000 women die each year, in the U.S., from breast cancer. It is believed that by the time breast cancer is detected, it has been developing for 8 or 10 years. The incidence of breast cancer for American women is 1 in 8. The African-American woman has a 1 in 4.5 chance of developing breast cancer as well as 2.2 times the relative risk for dying of the disease over her white counterpart — for uterine and cervical cancers the black woman also suffers more than twice the incidence than the white woman. Despite numerous media accounts linking breast cancer to genetic factors, it is also claimed that "70% of breast cancer patients have no risk factors" – this of course is absolutely contrary to what natural health advocates have determined in that probably 65% or more of cancer cases are directly result from multiple environmental exposures. Breast cancer also effects 1,400 men annually in the U.S., resulting in 260 fatalities.

Excess iron supplementation in the diet has been theorized as contributing to the cancer risk. More definite cancer risks within the food chain include pesticides, food additives, artificial sweeteners, estrogen-mimicking chemicals, animal fats, PCBs in food packaging, lack of fiber in the diet, food processing as well as hormones and steroids used in meat and dairy production.

Stroke

Stroke afflicts an estimated half-million persons each year in the United States with about 150,000 deaths occurring annually. Those who survive stroke usually are expected to live with some manner of permanent brain damage which includes paralysis. Until June 1996, there were no drugs available for emergency treatment for victims arriving at the hospital, leaving medical attendants to merely wait and see how much permanent damage would occur or even if the patient would live. Even then, the new drug which was approved by the U.S. Food and Drug Administration (FDA), tPA (marketed by San Francisco-based Genentech Inc. under the trade name Activase) has been shown to demonstrate horrific side effects such as "dangerous bleeding in the brain."

Stroke is triggered by plaque and cholesterol buildup in the blood vessels, pieces of which break off and migrate into the fine blood vessels of the brain creating blood clots which cut off oxygen to brain cells. Thus, in every sense, stroke is another obvious disease of improper diet — obvious to everyone except for the medical establishment and drug manufacturers.

One of the dangers of drugs prescribed to cut cholesterol was revealed in a study conducted at UC San Francisco in late 1995 which warned that "two broad classes of anti-cholesterol medications, the so-called statins and fibrates", had been shown to cause cancer when given to laboratory rats in high doses. These include industry-leaders lovastatin and gemfibrozil, marketed under the trade names Mevacor and Lopid. Particularly cited as cancer risks were hundreds of thousands of young and middle-aged adults without heart disease who were taking the drugs in response to only moderately elevated blood cholesterol levels and would be taking them for years.

Thus, the dietary resolution is undoubtedly the wisest method to deal with the higher-than-desired levels of blood cholesterol which have been most directly associated with stroke and other circulatory disorders.

Diabetes

Diabetes truly has become an 'American epidemic'. Diabetes is the inability of the body to adequately process sugar from carbohydrates and thus triggering the pancreas to secrete too much insulin to lower blood sugar level. In effect, diabetes is a malfunction of the endocrine system, the system within the body which manufactures hormones which trigger and regulate numerous body organ functions. What must be noted is that environmental factors, far more than genetic propensity, is likely the single greatest contributing factor for developing diabetes. Thus, when diabetes runs through a family, it most likely would only have begun only when the family came to America. I challenge the medical establishment to find widespread diabetes among Blacks in Africa as it is found in the so-called African-American.

A study conducted at the Picower Institute for Medical Research in Manhasset, NY, in June 1996 pointed out the danger of "browned foods", a tasty but toxic combination found in such delights as charbroiled steak with barbecue sauce, honey-glazed turkey and ham as well as cinnamon rolls. The combination of sugar, protein and high cooking temperatures created high concentrations of a "a toxic material called advanced glycated end products, or AGEs" which are believed prime causes for the "deadly complications of diabetes."

AGEs are even more deadly in persons with diabetes-induced kidney disease. Glue-like AGEs clog up the blood vessels, stiffening the arteries and leading to formation of plaque and clots – impeding the tiny pores that strip waste from the blood. Healthy people and diabetics in the study only excreted 30% of the AGEs they consumed while diabetics with kidney damage only excreted 5%, leaving 95% of the harmful toxins behind to clog up the body's organs.

The study, conducted by Dr. Helen Vlassara, should lead to "proper dietary guidelines" such as to avoid mixing sugars and proteins (a fundamental of Western diets, browned meats, barbecue, baked pastas and baked goods in particular – donuts, cakes, pastries, etc.), more steaming of cooked foods and less grilling, frying, oven-baking and the likes.

Nearly a million people in the U.S. are Type 1 diabetics (also known as juvenile diabetes) which require daily insulin injections to control excess blood sugar.

It is estimated that 14 to 16 million Americans suffer from Type 2 diabetes (also known as adult diabetes). Mainstream scientists, especially those within the highly questionable genetic research community, are quick to blame diabetes on genetic propensity, what they will rarely talk about is the grotesque amount of sugar, processed food and cholesterol consumed in the average American's diet as well as poor food-combining, such as the combination of sugars with proteins at high temperature which creates AGEs. Without a doubt, Americans consume the highest amount of these toxic foods per capita of any nation in history. In actuality, adult diabetes has been proven controllable by strict dietary regimen, exercise and herbs (the allopathic doctors would substitute their drugs for Nature's herbs).

Countering these Major Diseases

Chronic heart disease and stroke, like all circulatory disorders, are nearly completely manageable through diet. Keys to foregoing such problems are managing fat intake, balancing levels of "good" and "bad" cholesterol, lowering triglyceride levels, lowering blood pressure, drinking plenty of fluids, adding fiber to the diet, getting the proper nutrients and avoiding food dangers such as advanced glycated end products.

A Harvard University School of Public Health study in February 1996 monitored a group of 40,000 men for six years and "found that fatal and nonfatal heart attacks were 41% less common among men who ate more than 28 grams of fiber daily, compared with those who ate less than 13 grams." It should be noted that the average American consumes only 12 to 15 grams of fiber each day, half of the federal dietary recommendations of 25 grams. Yet in Uganda, which has very little incidence of heart disease and nearly no colon disease (colon cancer is the leading cancer killer in the U.S.), researchers have determined that the average daily intake of fiber is 70 grams. For Kenya this figure is 86 grams. Thus it should well be noted that a likely cause for the phenomenal rates of chronic disease among African-Americans would likely be related to their widespread adoption of the Western diet which his high in fat and low in fiber.

The healthy benefits of two types of fiber are notable for preventing heart disease. Soluble fibers are soft and gel-like when mixed with water. Soluble fiber lowers elevated blood cholesterol and thus reduces risk of heart disease. Insoluble fibers are crude, dense and chewy and do not break down in digestion. It has been shown that insoluble fiber provides the greatest reduction in heart attack risk. Some of the best foods for fiber include whole wheat bran, kidney beans, whole apples, peas, celery, bananas, broccoli and grapefruit. According to my own analysis of this critical research, I would suggest that people should attempt to include at least 50 grams of fiber into their daily diet. This is also key to losing weight, a key component of any healthy cardiovascular program. Fiber makes the body feel full – this combined with moderated exercise nutrient supplementation and fresh raw vegetables should make losing weight relatively easy.

High-fiber foods, vegetarianism, beta carotene, vitamins E and C, folic acid, omega-3 fatty acids from seafood, garlic, potassium – these are among the key nutritional requirements to prevent or manage heart disease and stave off stroke. Of course, all healthy lifestyles include plenty of exercise and stress management, certainly heart disease and stroke are no exception. Drinking plenty of water, at least 64 ounces per day, is also key to cardiac output (the amount of blood being pumped during each beat) which is vital to proper distribution of nutrients throughout the body and blood pressure balance. Dietary avoidance of heart disease and stroke requires long-term lifestyle modification and such a healthy nutritional regime cannot be implemented too early in life.

There are numerous dietary considerations when it comes to countering cancer. Key here is emphasis on prevention and this requires the instilling of habits early in life that are conducive to optimal health. Certain nutrients have shown strong cancer fighting properties. The group of vitamin nutrients called antioxidants stand out for their anti-cancer qualities. These include vitamins A, C and E as well as betacarotene. These can be found in orange and yellow-colored fruits and vegetables, dark green leafy vegetables and cruciferous vegetables, which includes broccoli, cabbage, Brussels sprouts, cauliflower and kohlrabi.

In addition, the chief cancer killer in the U.S., colon cancer, is nearly completely connected to the lack of fiber in the American diet. In Uganda, where fiber intake averages 70 grams a day, chronic colon disease is rare. The opposite is true for the U.S. citizen who consumes, on average, a mere

12 to 15 grams of fiber daily. Thus an obvious way to combat this major killer would be a dramatic increase in fiber intake, double the U.S. recommended daily allowance (RDA) of 25-35 grams per day.

Another key to the record rates of cancer in industrialized countries is the massive exposure to cancer-causing chemicals, carcinogens, many of which are increasingly inserted into the food chain. These include agricultural chemicals, synthetic hormones such as the milk-production stimulant bovine growth hormone (BGH or BST), antibiotics, food preservatives such as the deadly nitrites which make hot dogs, along with hormone-pesticide-antibiotic-treated milk, the worst foods on the market for cancer, and a plethora of long-chain complex molecules made from petrochemicals. These unnatural food additives have taken a deadly toll in the brief historical period in which they have been used.

The subject of hormone treated milk has become increasingly more critical as additional research on the effects of BGH becomes more widely available. BGH was approved by the U.S. Food and Drug Administration in 1985. Despite the best efforts of consumer watchdogs, the labeling of products which contain the growth hormone has been defeated by the agribusiness lobby. Resent research has linked the use of BGH to increases in the tumor-producing hormone insulin-like growth factor 1 (IGF-1). The increased presence of IGF-1, which is believed to be more concentrated in pasteurized milk and absorbed through the walls of the gut, has increased the risk in humans of breast, colon and other gastrointestinal cancers. Despite the banning of BGH in Europe, it is doubtful that the FDA will reverse its policy anytime soon and declare the synthetic hormone too dangerous for American consumption.

Barring any radical intervention from an outraged public, the rate of utilization of this type of carcinogenic chemistry will only increase due to the greed and avarice of increasingly-dominant corporations and agribusiness. The major chemical manufacturers have also been grossly negligent in conducting the necessary studies to determine the long-term ill effects of widespread use of their products. Thus we can see efforts by manufacturers' organizations and political lobbying groups to thwart and undermine environmental standards which would curtail agricultural chemical usage.

The most health-producing foods are the most natural and unadulterated, thus making the anti-cancer diet readily available to all who would just demonstrate the will to show nutritional consciousness. Yet often even basically healthy foods can be prepared in a way as to make them carcinogenic. A recent article appeared in the Los Angeles Times, entitled "Way Meat Is Cooked Linked to Cancer". In it the National Cancer Institute (NCI) "suggests that cooking meat too long – and at too high a temperature – increases the risk of cancer", as well as pointing out the dangers of carcinogens in fats (pan drippings) used in gravy. The animal protein known as creatinine was shown in the NCI study to become carcinogenic when heated to high temperatures. High-temperature cooking also negatively affects fruits and vegetables.

Chapter 2 – What Is Making You So Crazy?

The subject of meat consumption linked to brain disease has firmly come to the fore with the issue of 'mad cow' disease. While scientists debate whether it is due to a mysterious prion or a virus, health-conscious advocates and nutritionists are using the scandal to point out numerous disadvantages of the typical animal-based Western diet as well as the unscrupulous manner in which the meat-producing industry is manufacturing its product.

Specifically, it is theorized that 'mad cow' disease results from contaminated animal feed which has been 'fortified' with ground-up intestines, brains, spinal cords, bones and other parts from cows, chickens and sheep – in effect turning herbivores into cannibalistic carnivores.

With 'mad cow' disease (also known as bovine spongiform encephalopathy – BSE), which is being linked to a correspondingly similar brain disorder in humans known as Creutzfeldt-Jakob disease, the symptoms are attributed to microscopic holes in the brain.

Direct and indirect negative effects of certain other dietary habits on the mental state is well documented. Among the more obvious are: the role of sugar in hyperactivity among children as well as emotional problems among all ages, food allergies spawning learning disabilities and agricultural chemicals linked to neurological impairment.

Sugar has been referred to as the "most abused drug on the planet" and the damaging affects of this non-food has been well publicized. Sugar comes in many forms beyond the common highly processed version with which most of us are most familiar. Sucrose, glucose, fructose, maltose, dextrose, lactose, galactose, levulose – these are all different manifestations of the same thing...sugar! Unprocessed, or "low-tech" sugars maintain their natural stores of minerals and vitamins along with other valuable nutrients and are metabolized by the body better than "high-tech" sugars.

White sugar has been proven to be damaging to the body, impeding the digestion of other nutrients, contributing to a host of chronic diseases and impeding the immune system, in addition to the mental disruptions which we have all heard about. Substitutes for common white sugar, which all nutritionists agree should be eliminated from the diet, include: pure maple syrup, maple sugar, barley malt syrup, brown rice syrup, fruit juice concentrate, dried cane juice, honey, date sugar and granular fruit sweetener.

Chemical sugar substitutes such as NutriSweet, aspartame and saccharine, have demonstrated carcinogenic, or cancer-causing, effects and thus should be avoided by every means possible (many so-called "diet" sweets and colas contain these chemicals).

Nourishment for an Old, Tired Brain

There have been numerous studies that have demonstrated the beneficial effects of four herbs on the mental processes:

- **Ginkgo Biloba** – has achieved widespread acclaim for reversing "decreased mental capacity due to a physical disability or advancing years", increasing oxygen to the brain, delaying the early stages of Alzheimer's disease, "making people over age 60 feel more alert, attentive, sociable and less moody after just one to two months", improving immediate short-term memory, attention span and quickening perception. In increased the effects of ginkgo biloba are said to be quick-acting.

- **Panax Ginseng** – another favorite brain herb contains ginsenoside compounds that increase brain neurotransmitter activity along with protein synthesis. This popular herb is said to improve concentration and intellectual performance, therefore decreasing mistakes along with increasing reading speed.

- **Siberian Ginseng** – this cousin of Panax ginseng has reported the same effects along with certain other beneficial results when given to patients diagnosed as senile or suffering mental disorders from atherosclerosis. This herb is also recommended for women suffering from symptoms of pre-menopause and menopause. Benefits are said to include balancing hormone production in the adrenal glands, thus easing hormone-induced stress, along with relieving the fatigue and irritability of menopause.

- **Gotu Kola** – this popular herb from India has widespread acclaim for its ability to have "energized and preserved the brain cells of anyone who took it". Clinical studies have shown that those who took gotu kola scored higher on standardized intelligence tests.

Additional beneficial claims for this herb have included improved behavioral patterns for "mentally challenged children", increased mental alertness as well as feelings of relaxation and calmness.

In addition, studies have shown that vitamin B6 can affect serotonin levels in the brains of children, providing a more desirable alternative to the Ritalin which is currently being prescribed to hundreds of thousands of schoolchildren and young adults who have been mis-labeled as attention deficit disorder (ADD), hyperactivity and other dubious diagnoses of learning disabilities.

In actuality, the learning disabilities for which the medical-pharmaceutical, psychiatric and educational establishments are so quick to proscribe drug solutions, can quite likely be resolved by merely investigating the possibility of food allergies in the child (also consider that the same reactions do occur among adults). The greatest offenders which create conflict within a child's blood/brain chemistry include: sugar (candy bars, gum, soda, cookies, ice cream, etc.), artificial food colors and flavors, MSG, dairy products, oranges, corn, chocolate, eggs and wheat. Thus elimination diets, where single foods are isolated as possible triggers for hyperactivity or other allergic reaction, can be useful to indicate just which food items are causing problems in the affected child.

Among nutrient supplements which research has shown beneficial toward creating the proper blood/brain chemistry, are large doses of vitamin B6, other vitamins (A, B complex, C, D and E) along with such minerals as calcium, magnesium, chromium and zinc. One study which appeared in the British medical journal The Lancet circa

1987 noted a 9-point increase in verbal intelligence among children who were receiving a broad multivitamin-mineral supplement over another group which was not supplemented.

Chapter 3 – Sexual Dysfunction and Infertility

A Crisis of the Developed World

In recent decades, scientific research has raised an alarm over growing evidence that widespread use of industrial chemicals, pesticides, herbicides and household chemicals has created serious reproductive problems within the industrialized nations. Chief among these reproductive problems include:

- European studies which indicate a nearly 50% drop in average sperm count among men in industrialized countries, falling from an average of 122 million cells per milliliter to 66 million cells per milliliter along with a 19% drop in semen volume.

- A rise in testicular cancer in developed countries, increasing approximately 300% in the past three decades.

- Links between exposures to endocrine disrupting chemicals (EDCs) to epidemics of endometriosis, breast, uterine and cervical cancers within women in industrialized countries.

- High rates of gender-mutation among animals, birds and fish found in areas with high concentrations of EDCs especially in Lake Apopka, Florida, the Great Lakes region and the Columbia River.

- Alarming numbers of babies within the developed countries showing evidence of reproductive malfunction such as undescended testicles, hermaphroditic genital formations, crossed male-female DNA and sexual organs, as well as sexual-neurological malfunction – all evidence supporting a biophysical basis for homosexuality.

- The unprecedented decline in fertility among women and men in the countries where exposure to EDCs is greatest.

- An explosive growth in the industry of invitro fertilization, test-tube conception methods, artificial insemination, surrogate parenting, and other substitutes for natural, unimpeded parenting.

Food Contaminants Inhibit Reproduction

Without a doubt, one of the major routes by which these destructive EDCs are entering our bodies is through an increasingly contaminated food chain – a food delivery system that is an evolutionarily recent development.

Agricultural chemicals are suspected to be the chief source of chemical-induced reproductive disorders. The suspect family of chemicals, endocrine disrupters, have become so widely used that we are virtually surrounded by a "sea of estrogens" and estrogenic chemicals. This is at the heart of the epidemic of infertility.

It cannot be overemphasized that the chief source of EDCs in the food chain is agricultural chemicals. These include dozens of pesticides (the number of which will likely increase many-fold as better designed research studies into the long-term effects of pesticide combinations are conducted), numerous herbicides, synthetic hormones such as bovine growth hormone (BGH, BST), and naturally-occurring animal hormones – all of which have permeated the animal-protein-based, chemically-saturated Western diet.

In addition, polychlorinated biphenyls (PCBs), which are widely used in food packaging and water bottles, is also known to be an endocrine disrupting chemical which leaches into the products that this packaging contains. What becomes even more troubling, tiny traces of these pollutants may not demonstrate direct deleterious effects but can become devastating when in combination with trace amounts of other endocrine disrupters.

In fact, recent research into the endocrine-disrupting effect of chemical pollutants has indicated that combining pesticides has shown to increase estrogenic potency from 160 to 1,600 times. Tulane University endocrinologist John A. McLachlan claimed, in a LA Times article June 7, 1996, "Instead of 1 plus 1 equaling 2, we found that 1 plus 1 equals a thousandfold. We expected interactions, but we were surprised they were so strong." His research on polychlorinated biphenyls (PCBs) showed the same synergistic affect, increasing estrogenic potency from 5 to 7 times when 2 PCBs were combined. It is believed that there are about 209 different PCBs in use.

Foods known to be particularly loaded with EDCs include: grapes, apples, strawberries, bottle and tap water (especially ground water from agricultural regions), dairy products, animal fats and vegetables upon which the highest amounts of agricultural chemicals, pesticides and herbicides, hormones and steroids are used.

Obesity has been undeniably linked to birth defects, notably neural tube defects such as spina bifida and anencephaly (where a baby is born missing portions of the brain). Other dietary links to birth defects include diabetes and folic acid deficiencies (vitamin B12). Key to this obesity connection is the way obesity interrupts nutrient absorption in the stomach thus making it difficult for the body to obtain key vitamins, minerals, amino acids and enzymes which are necessary for proper metabolism. Thus, we must recognize that pregnant women need to have a strict nutritional regime and avoid the trap of irrational cravings during pregnancy for high-sugar junk foods which is merely silly mythology.

Chapter 4 – Other Diet-Disease Connections

Common Ailments with Common Causes

I make no pretense that this book can cover the entire spectrum of disorders and diseases for which food solutions would handily work. Yet, because there are so many ailments with chronic inflammation as their root cause, a little bit of really good advice can go a long way toward prevention. By settling upon an anti-inflammation nutritional lifestyle, one can assure themselves that they will experience much better health than is average within this society.

Let us look into a few more of these common ailments for which our nutritional strategies can have a huge, positive impact.

Arthritis

—The CDC reported in June 1996 that adults might be able to reduce their risk of arthritis by controlling their weight. "Men who are overweight or underweight are more likely to suffer...than adults of normal weight... Obese women are at risk, but underweight women apparently aren't." This was reported in the *LA Times* June 17, 1996.

Hypertension

– This is a disorder which affects an estimated 23% of the U.S. population and affects Blacks at even greater numbers. Hypertension, or high blood pressure, is linked to other illnesses, worsening already-bad conditions like heart attack, stroke, heart failure, kidney failure and other problems. In nearly 90% of all cases, diet, food supplementation and lifestyle modification can control hypertension. Common symptoms of hypertension include morning headaches, ringing in the ears, unexplained dizziness, nose bleeds, depression, blurred vision, unprovoked tension and fainting spells.

Conditions which significantly affect the risk for developing hypertension include obesity and cholesterol. High blood pressure, along with the prescription drugs used to "control" it, is one of the key factors limiting our enjoyment of our senior years. In early 1995, scientific advisors to the FDA issued an alert on one type of blood pressure medication, nifedipine, one of a class of so-called calcium channel blocks sold under the brand names of Aldalat and Procardia, which had been linked to a tripling of patient death rates and a 60% increased risk of heart attack. Blood pressure medications are associated with impotence among men on the drugs, a common side affect that negatively impacts the quality of life.

Key dietary factors in overcoming or preventing hypertension are: controlling our consumption of salt, proper intake of minerals including potassium, calcium and magnesium, dietary fiber, plenty of omega-3 fatty acids (referred to in one article as "nature's Teflon"), avoiding "bad" fats and alcohol, and getting sufficient water intake.

Immune Deficiencies

– Those who are familiar with the Conscious Rasta Perspective should well know by now that I fundamentally do not believe that there is an "AIDS-causing virus" and believe there is no proof that the so-called human immunodeficiency virus (HIV) is destroying the immune systems of millions of persons around the world as is being claimed throughout the media [re: Conscious Rasta Report Vol. 3, No. 1: ***AIDS EXPOSED***].

In contrast, following the lead of hundreds of doctors, scientists and researchers, which includes 5 Nobel Prize-winning researchers, I have come to conclude that the immune deficiencies we are witnessing, no matter what level they are actually occurring, stem from the negative effects of environmental influences such as epidemics of drug use (legal and otherwise), malnutrition, overmedication, stress, food allergies and toxic overload from a myriad of daily exposures to chemicals, pollutants, pesticides, food additives or other unnatural substances. This appears to have been confirmed by an article which appeared in the *Los Angeles Times* on May 13, 1996, written by Marla Cone, entitled "**Human Immune Systems May Be Pollution Victims.**" In that well-researched article, Ms. Cone noted the immune damage, linked to environmental toxins, which were permeating the food chain, affecting fish, animals, and humans alike. She specifically cited breast milk, seafood, contaminated water, food and air as the likely vehicles for substances which were so negatively impacting immune systems of those affected.

Thus a nutritional regimen for combating immune deficiency would be first and foremost an avoidance of such toxic influences in our food and water. This would include such likely culprits as dairy products, fried foods, frozen and canned foods, processed foods, animal, fish and fowl – "all dead food produces dead cells", this according to a broadsheet put out by the Natural Living Institute of Los Angeles.

Foods to eat would include garlic, antioxidant vitamins, echinecea, goldenseal, aloe vera, wheatgrass juice, cayenne pepper, carrots, spinach, beets, cucumber along with other foods and herbs which have demonstrated blood cleansing, healing or immune system building functions.

Avoiding Contaminated Food & Water

One area which few parents consider as potentially hazardous to their children is the risk of contaminated food in the schools. A recent *Associated Press* article, entitled "**Probe of N.Y, School Cafeterias Finds Roaches, Mice**", brings to mind the absolute necessity to question "Who's going to police the schools when it comes to our children's proper nutrition?" This article not only detailed filthy conditions breeding roaches and rats within school cafeterias but also referred to disturbing conditions such as when a "teenager said he had eaten a half-cooked hamburger that he called the 'murder burger special.'" Now if teenagers in New York have that kind of perception of the food they are being served in the schools, is it possible that the problem throughout the nation could be as bad or even worse?

We have well noted throughout this report of the damage being done to our food through pesticides (the probable chemical resolution to the cockroach problem noted in the previous paragraph would be far worse than any contamination by creeping pests), herbicides and a wide host of industrial chemicals. Thus, even the careless vegetarian might be susceptible to many of the same damaging effects of contaminated diet. Where can one turn to resolve the problem of consuming these unwanted byproducts of the food production industry? Is eating vegan a healthy alternative?

The single solution to this dilemma is in the word organic. Organic vegetables and fruits are deliberately grown using no distilled petrochemicals and other unnatural substances. Organic fruits and veggies might occasionally have bug bites in them, may not have the strong visual appeal of waxed fruits, cucumbers, peppers, and the likes. But without exception organic produce tastes better and is loaded with more useful nutrients than non-organic produce.

Unfortunately for most urban dwellers, access to organic products – which includes not only fruits and vegetables but fabrics, household supplies, building supplies and other materials – getting these products is more difficult, more expensive and requires more concentrated effort to conduct the proper shopping research. Key to this solution is establishing proper routines for acquiring our food and water.

The ideal solution for organic produce is to have one's own garden. Increasingly, among progressive families, even in the non-conducive urban environment, planting gardens and studying the various methodologies which make up organic farming is becoming the solution of choice. An excellent array of organic gardening magazines and books (including my own The Organic Gardener) can guide the backyard agriculturist with a wealth of knowledge on how to establish this wonderful source of organic produce.

There is also an explosion in businesses catering to the demand for vegan, non-contaminated foodstuffs. Thus in most major urban centers one can find organic produce in dedicated healthfood stores, cooperative buyers networks and farmers markets (not all farmers supplying these markets use organic techniques so it is necessary to inquire directly about the use of chemicals from each particular vender).

The Community Alliance With Family Farmers publishes the excellent National Organic Directory, an impressive 370-page directory of the burgeoning organic industry throughout the U.S. The directory is a wealth of knowledge listing farmers, wholesalers, suppliers, support businesses, certification groups and resource groups as well as providing up-to-date research articles on various subjects related to organic production. In addition it provides lists of magazines, newsletters & reports, books, directories and catalogues which will supplement your expertise on all matters organic.

The Community Alliance with Family Farmers can be contacted at: (800)852-3832 or e-mailed at: <caff@igc.apc.org>. The 1996 directory is their 13th edition of this outstanding publication.

Another key concern is the widespread contamination of water supplies with the very same chemicals, and others of equal toxicity, which are causing the devastation of the food supply. Big city water suppliers have made no great secret of the fact that urban water supplies contain a long list of chemical and organic elements (in this case, organic substances are undesirable – notably human and animal waste residues), harmful pathogens such as e. coli and cryptosporidiosis, as well as deliberately-induced contamination such as , and fluoridation.

Thus a feasible solution would be to obtain water that has been filtered for these very types of contaminants. Unfortunately the billion-dollar bottled-water delivery system has utilized deceptive marketing practices which allows them to sell water which is often not much better than that which comes from the tap. The plastic bottle which much of the drinking water is packaged in is itself a source of gender-bending PCBs.

An ideal solution for this would be a "point of use" water filter. Point of use devices filter your drinking water right at the point where you want to use it yourself. Yet, herein lies another problem in that marketers of water filtration systems use misleading advertising techniques to make one think that taste alone is a proper measure of drinking water quality. Thus, water which "tastes sparkling clean" with no obvious chlorine smell or taste could likely still be laden with chemical pollutants, heavy metals, microorganisms, and other food-borne dangers.

The highest quality water filter on the market features a solid-block carbon filter instead of the lesser-efficient granular carbon filter. Industry standards vary widely, with some popular models filtering to 20 microns while other models are filtering down to .2 microns. This is a ten-fold difference, so one should be cautious when a $20 filter promises to deliver the same results as a $300 filter or others, such as reverse osmosis, which can run into the thousands of dollars.

A fair amount of study will be necessary to find the most efficient water filter to fulfill your own needs. By all means, it is well worth the time and expense required to obtain for yourself and your children the highest quality of water available – and then to ensure that you drink your eight eight-ounce glasses of pure water daily!

Chapter 5 – Fighting Food Addiction and Obesity

Among that segment of the population which struggles to shed excess weight, each month brings new hopes of drug breakthroughs, miracle diets, incredible claims, surgical techniques and fad diets of every level of credibility. Yet it is often not how much we eat but what we eat that triggers obesity. According to an article which appeared in U.S. News & World Report, January 8, 1996, entitled "Are You Too Fat?", there are certain foods which are the favorites for men and women who consider themselves overweight.

The most popular foods for obese men and women are: 1) steaks and roasts, 2) ice cream and frozen desserts, 3) chicken or turkey (not fried), 4) doughnuts, cookies and cake, 5) bread, rolls and crackers, 6) pasta, 7) fish (baked, broiled, canned), 8) pizza, 9) cheese, 10) potatoes (not fried), 11) candy and chocolate.

One of the more disturbing developments of recent is the U.S. Food and Drug Administration's (FDA) approval of a new synthetic fat marketed under the trade name Olestra. The fat substitute, marketed by Procter & Gamble, is said to cause a number of serious digestive problems including nutrient depletion, diarrhea, cramps, incontinence, bloating and "'anal leakage' where the liquid product seeps out, staining the underwear". Michael Jacobson, executive director of the Center for Science in the Public Interest, which is backed by the American Public Health Association, stated in the *Los Angeles Times* June 13, 1996, that "the three test cities [where Olestra-related products are being test-marketed] are rapidly becoming the diarrhea capitals of America." Opponents have contested the introduction of such synthetic fat substitutes for nearly a decade. Despite such reports of negative side effects, the FDA and food manufacturers stand by this product. The public has yet to really register its acceptance as Olestra is just now being used on such products as potato chips and corn chips from Frito-Lay.

Another aspect of "voodoo dieting" is the endless pursuit of prescription solutions for obesity. Among the latest prescriptions gaining popularity within upscale circles is the so-called Fen-Phen program. This regimen calls for the combination of two prescription drugs. Fenfluramine is said to raise levels of serotonin, brain hormones which are linked to decreased appetite, increased feelings of fullness and mood enhancement. Phentermine, it is claimed, works in the brain and releases noradrenaline, preventing uptake of adrenaline and giving a high feeling. This new drug-diet fad is utilized primarily by the financially well-off due to fees ranging upward from $600 at UCLA for six months of drugs preceded by a battery of clinical diagnostic tests. Side effects include pulmonary hypertension, depression, insomnia, fatigue, diarrhea, headaches, jitters, blood pressure increase, a "feeling of spaciness" and short term memory loss in some patients.

Advertisements and news reports are replete with such accounts of weight-reduction schemes, yet little emphasis is given to several simple rules of nutrition and metabolism. Common throughout such fad diets is emphasis on some product which the promoter serves to be the exclusive supplier thereof, cursory acknowledgment to the weight-reduction benefits of fresh fruits and vegetables along with exercise, and generous use of mind control techniques and propaganda to hook potential consumers.

In reality, weight management requires just a few simple rules which, if followed, would probably make losing weight much less of a painful sacrifice and more of a life-enhancing process.

According to my own research (and realize that I am not speaking from experience as my weight has increased only about ten pounds since graduating high school 23 years ago), a weight-reduction program should be based upon the following simple rules:

- Five to nine servings of fresh organic fruits and vegetables daily, preferably raw to preserve vital digestive enzymes.

- Avoid eating out; fast-food and restaurant dining contribute to eating an excess of empty calories.

- Supplementation of vitamins, minerals, amino acids and enzymes (the basic four nutrient categories which humans require).

- Consumption of a minimum of 50 grams of fiber daily (double the U.S. RDA of 25 grams/daily), increasing fiber should correspondingly increase weight loss.

- Drinking a minimum of 8 eight-ounce glasses of pure water daily, even more if your weight is more than 30 pounds over your ideal.

- Brisk physical activity for at least 30 minutes each day.

- Periods each day devoted to meditation as well as self-education on health-related issues.

An emphasis on nutritional education cannot be understated because when it comes down to the means by which one acquires fruits and vegetables, which supplements to take and in what ratios, which foods have the specific nutrients necessary, etc., one will have to be vigilant in monitoring one's progress.

In effect, the pursuit of knowledge about proper nutrition places one in a healthy mental state where each and every opportunity to make correct food choices becomes empowering. With such a holistic health consciousness it becomes little of a chore to bypass foods which are obviously detrimental to one's well being such as meat, dairy products, junk foods and sugar. I find that it also helps to associate with those who share your interest in nutritional matters and rely upon each other as reinforcement for maintaining discipline.

Chapter 6 – Eat to Age Gracefully

The key to reaching a kinder and gentler senior stage of life is to have lifelong habits of good nutrition, exercise, and stress management. Thus, to have good health in the senior years begin this type of beneficial lifestyle while as young as possible.

Too often we witness the tragedy of one such as Ella Fitzgerald, this century's greatest female improvisational singer and one of the greatest musical talents of all times. Ella, because of the lifestyle of her celebrity, had a long bout with poor health, specifically diabetes, which tried to rob her of her productive senior years. Fortunately for jazz lovers, the worst physical conditions could not steal the talent, eloquence, and grace with which the Creator blessed Ella Fitzgerald. Nonetheless we are only left to wonder what would have been the case had she not suffered for decades from diminished eyesight and eventually from amputation of her legs due to complications from diabetes?

Thus, from breast milk for the newborn to easily-digestible fruits and vegetables in our senior years, we would be best to be diligent and cautious about just how we are going to respect nutrition. The years from our teens until our forties, during which we perceive ourselves invulnerable to dietary excess (unless of course we have already been diagnosed from some chronic condition such as juvenile diabetes, obesity, asthma, etc.) – this is when we need to be concerned just as much as when our young bodies are rapidly growing or when those Autumn years begin to make themselves known.

Many of us can look at our parents or grandparents and get some hint as to what our own senior years will present. I don't adhere to the myth of genetic predisposition to chronic disease which is so often presented in the media and in medical advertising. One way to show the folly of this type of genetic mislabeling is to compare African-Americans to their cousins on the Motherland. Chronic disorders such as heart disease, cancer and diabetes simply aren't prevalent in Africa as they are among Blacks in America. So it becomes obvious that there must be some other sort of environmental influence that is causing the damage here. I am convinced it is the result of the stress of racism combined with poor nutrition and exposure to toxic chemicals. Thus, to the best of our abilities we must establish control over these factors and seek to change the reality of the poor health which has overtaken us here.

Without a doubt, from our middle years until the end of our lives, we need to be concerned and focused on what foods we need to be consuming and in what quantities. Throughout this report I have championed the simple rules of good nutrition – 5 to 9 servings of fresh, organic fruits and vegetables daily, vitamins, minerals, amino acids and enzyme supplementation, high-fiber diet, pure drinking water, avoiding toxic foods and consuming foods which have the least amount of processing possible.

To age gracefully certain foods should be avoided like the disease-causing plagues that they are. Included among these, and certainly not limited to this short list are: white sugar and many sugar substitutes (all artificial sweeteners), bleached flour, hydrogenated vegetable oils, meats along with animal byproducts such as lard and gelatins, shellfish, eggs, dairy products, food additives (such as monosodium glutamate (MSG), preservatives like nitrites and sulfur dioxide, etc.), fried foods, candies, sodas, canned foods and most any other highly-processed food as well as contaminated water. Again, this list is not complete, but strict avoidance of the kind of disease-causing foods which are on this short list will likely add productive years to our lives.

The Road Forward

I have so much enjoyed doing the research for this article that I wish I could continue to write on this subject of Food for Life indefinitely. Most certainly, I will be continuing food and nutritional research for the rest of my life. During the weeks it took to compose this text I have already made significant changes in my own dietary habits like cutting the last vestiges of animal products from my diet such as eggs, significantly upgrading my daily fiber intake and eating more raw, organic fruits and vegetables each day.

Dr. Joel Wallach (a.k.a. the mineral doctor), nutritionist-researcher, 1991 Nobel Prize nominee, and veteran of tens of thousands of autopsies, has published an audio cassette called "Dead Doctors Don't Lie." He points out that the average lifespan of doctors in the U.S. is 58 years and lectures on the value of minerals, an under-appreciated nutrient. Of 90 nutrients our body requires, Dr. Wallach identifies 60 minerals which are critical to maintaining health, adding years to our lives (Wallach travels the world documenting populations whose members routinely live to between 120 and 140 years. Two major themes of his presentation are 1) that the practices of mainstream doctors are absolutely scandalous, driven by money and responsible for an admitted 300,000 deaths-per-year from simple mistakes, and 2) of the three types of mineral supplements sold, colloidal minerals are best absorbed in our bodies. Dr. Wallach's research links most causes of death in humans and animals, with mineral deficiencies. He states the absorption rate of standard metalized minerals, as about 3%, the rest excreted by the body. Chelated minerals, which are bound to amino acids, are 40% absorbed. 97% of colloidal minerals are absorbed. Colloids are extremely small particles, thousands of times smaller than blood cells, which are charged with a negative ion and suspended in liquids. Based upon the wonderful, logical info on this cassette tape, I'm glad I made recent decision to use colloidal minerals as a daily supplement along with vitamins, fiber, garlic and herbs.

If I could wave a magic wand and produce an immediate change in the condition of the sufferers of the world, it would certainly be to instill the kind of information on nutrition of which I have written in this article. Yet, life is not about magic wands and instant gratification. The fact is that the masses are highly resistant to this type of life-enhancing information and usually one must beg an audience to take this type of research seriously. Nonetheless, I'm sure that the data presented herein will have some sort of lasting effect on those who read it, either on their personal lives or on their abilities as teachers to better present the already-positive information that they possess. When we advocate for holistic health present our case, it should be noted that we are talking about real revolution – a change in thought, action, and circumstance. Before we can talk about monumental social or political changes, we had better be able to look at ourselves, at our own bodies, and make sure that we aren't just trying to divert attention from more immediate problems which we are unable to confront.

I must confess, that my health is pretty good. I have never had to deal with obesity or any of the chronic diseases which I have herein written about. I have been to a doctor and dentist for minor problems only twice in over 15 years. Thus, I either am writing about things of which I know very little – or about a subject which I have already mastered in my own personal affairs.

Perhaps the most important point of this article is that nutritional research is exciting, very rewarding and a significant step toward overcoming some of the most persistent and destructive social conditions which affect the world. When we change our attitude and begin to view every meal as either a healing session or a "dance with the devil" over our long-term health, then we can commit ourselves to how we will experience the latter stages of life. I challenge the reader: Which way will it be – when you become a senior citizen, or mzee, will you be robbed of some your most productive years because of poor health or will you grow old gracefully?

This question must be answered by us individually and for our children, today and every day of our lives. Food is for Life!

References for Food For Life

1)   ASSESSING ENVIRONMENTAL HEALTH RISKS by Ann Misch, from State of the World 1994, Worldwatch Institute

2)   EATING WELL THROUGH THE DECADES by Colleen Dunn Bates, Vegetarian Times, March 1996

3)   BGH LINKED TO CANCER IN HUMANS by Amy O'Conner, Vegetarian Times, March 1996

4)   BLUE-CHIP FOODS, by Winifred Yu, Vegetarian Times, June 1996

5)   WHY YOUR BODY NEEDS WATER by Vince & Yolanda, The Challenger, December 6, 1995

6)   SMALL TRACES OF POLLUTANTS CAN AFFECT BRAIN DEVELOPMENT, SURVEY FINDS by Robert Lee Hotz, Los Angeles Times, May 31, 1996

7)   STUDIES LINK MOTHERS' OBESITY TO BABIES' NEURAL TUBE DEFECTS by Thomas H. Maugh II, Los Angeles Times, April 10, 1996

8)   WAY MEAT IS COOKED LINKED TO CANCER from the Associated Press, Los Angeles Times, April 23, 1996

9)   46 PESTICIDE BRANDS TO NO LONGER BE AVAILABLE IN STATE from Associated Press, Los Angeles Times, May 24, 1996

10)   MAJOR CLUE TO TYPE 2 DIABETES' CAUSES FOUND by Thomas H. Maugh II, Los Angeles Times, May 31, 1996

11)   MAD COW DISEASE: IS IT A PRION OR A VIRUS? by Kenneth Chang, Los Angeles, Times, May 26, 1996

12)   PROBE OF N.Y. SCHOOL CAFETERIAS FINDS ROACHES, MICE from Associated Press, Los Angeles Times

13)   ADDING FIBER CUTS HEART ATTACK RISK, STUDY FINDS by Terence Monmaney, Los Angeles Times Feb 14, 1996

14)   DOGGING OLESTRA, Los Angeles Times, June 13, 1996

15)   SLIM HOPES by Kathleen Doheny, Los Angeles, Times June 11, 1996

16)   HAZARDS: BROWNED FOOD MAY CARRY HARMFUL TOXINS by Thomas H. Maugh II, Los Angeles Times, June 10, 1996

17)   STUDY WARNS OF EFFECTS OF MIXED CHEMICALS by Marla Cone, Los Angeles Times, June 7, 1996

18)   NATIONAL ORGANIC DIRECTORY published by Community Alliance With Family Farmers, 1996, (800)852-3832

19)   GENENTECH CLOT-DISSOLVING DRUG GETS FEDERAL APPROVAL from Times Wire Services, Los Angeles Times, June 19, 1996

20)   ARTHRITIS LINKED TO WEIGHT, STUDY FINDS from Times Staff and Wire Reports, Los Angeles Times, June 17, 1996

21)   THE NEW GROLIER MULTIMEDIA ENCYCLOPEDIA from Multimedia PC, 1993, electronic listing under "heart diseases"

22)   EATING WELL THROUGH THE DECADES by Coleen Dunn Bates, Vegetarian Times, March 1996

23)   FOOD SUPPLEMENTS FOR HIGH BLOOD PRESSURE by Dr. James Scala, published by Bruce Miller Enterprises Inc., 1989

24)   HEALING AIDS NATURALLY, from a broadsheet published by the Natural Living Institute, 1749 La Cienega Blvd., Los Angeles, Ca 90035, (213)737-1123

25)   HUMAN IMMUNE SYSTEMS MAY BE POLLUTION VICTIMS by Marla Cone, Los Angeles Times, May 13, 1996

26)   'TIMMY, YOU'RE DRIVING ME CRAZY!' by William G. Crook, MD, Better Nutrition, December 1988

27)   CANCER PREVENTION: THE DIRTY DOZEN, (12 most cancer-causing products) Vegetarian Times, March 1996

28)   NEW FAKE FAT IS SAFE, FEDERAL ADVISERS DECIDE by Marlene Cimons, Los Angeles Times, November 18, 1995

29)   THE FACTS ON FIBER by Gene A. Spiller, DSc., PhD, Veggie Life, May 1996

30)   STOP SINGING THE SUGAR BLUES (author, source and publication date unknown)

31)   BOOST YOUR BRAIN POWER by Kathi Keville, Vegetarian Times, March 1996

32)   A WOMAN'S MEDICINE CHEST: TEN HERBS FOR WOMEN'S UNIQUE NEEDS by Judith Benn Hurley, Vegetarian Times, July 1996

33)   ARE YOU TOO FAT? by Traci Watson and Corinna Wu, U.S. News & World Report, January 8, 1996

34)   DEAD DOCTORS DON'T LIE : LEARN WHY THE AVERAGE LIFE SPAN OF AN MD IS ONLY 58 YEARS by Dr. Joel Wallach, B.S., D.V.M.,N.D., 1991 Nobel Prize Nominee - Medicine, 1995

Chapter 7 – Eat to Beat Cancer & Heart Disease

As much as two-thirds of heart disease and cancer can be attributed to bad diet habits. Nutritionists recommend at least five servings of fruit and vegetables each day yet only ten percent of us do so. Key nutrients called antioxidants show great value for ridding the body of poisons which have been linked to cancer. Study the following information carefully. It could very well save your life! – Keidi Obi Awadu

Book Review: The Antioxidant Pocket Counter

Much of the information that I've compiled in this chapter is referenced from ***THE ANTIOXIDANT POCKET COUNTER: A Guide to the Essential Nutrients That Help Fight Cancer and Heart Disease***, by Gail L. Becker, R.D., 1993, Random House.

Antioxidants are substances found naturally in the body which react with foreign elements to neutralize their potentially harmful effects. Specifically, antioxidants protect cells from damage caused by free radicals. Free radicals are highly reactive chemical substances that are produced during oxidation, the body's natural process for burning fuel for energy.

Free radicals provide some beneficial functions such as assisting germ-killing cells in fighting off certain types of bacteria. However, they are also caused by exposure to hazardous elements such as cigarette smoke, carcinogens, pollution, environmental toxins, exhaust fumes, radiation, excessive sunlight, and certain medications.

Vitamins C, E and beta carotene have been noted for their antioxidant benefits and as such have been shown to reduce the risk of cancer, heart disease, arthritis, cataracts, and conditions due to aging.

Vitamin A is necessary for vision, reproduction, growth, and healthy skin, hair, and body tissues. Much of the vitamin A found in our bodies is obtained from foods high in beta carotene, which is converted into vitamin A.

Beta carotene is found in yellow-orange colored fruits and vegetables, such as cantaloupe and carrots, and is present in green leafy vegetables such as spinach. Beta carotene has been shown to provide protective effects against certain forms of cancer, including lung, stomach, colon, prostate, and cervical cancer. It also has benefits for protection against cataracts, immune disease, skin disorders, strokes and heart disease.

Top sources for beta carotene are carrots, sweet potatoes, pumpkin, cantaloupe, leafy greens (spinach, kale, mustard greens, collard greens, Swiss chard, etc.), winter squash, apricots, mangoes, persimmon and broccoli.

Vitamin C is useful for many body functions including enhancing iron absorption, producing collagen (for skin integrity), wound healing and stimulating the immune system. It also may play an important role in preventing heart disease, lowering blood pressure, raising levels of "good" cholesterol and preventing oxidation of "bad" cholesterol. Vitamin C also aids in the prevention of certain forms of cancer, including oral, stomach, esophageal, pancreatic, lung and rectal cancers.

Top sources of vitamin C include melons, citrus fruits, peppers, leafy greens, strawberries, tropical fruits (papaya, kiwi and mangoes), cruciferous vegetables (broccoli, cauliflower, Brussels sprouts, kohlrabi and cabbage), tomatoes, sweet potatoes and berries.

Vitamin E is believed to reduce the risk of stroke, heart disease and degenerative disorders such as cataracts, cancer (including stomach, bladder, breast, colon, rectum and lung cancers), and immune-function disorders.

Top sources of vitamin E are seeds, nuts, vegetable oils, mayonnaise, wheat germ, leafy greens, seafood, avocados, mangoes, whole grains and cereals.

Dietary fiber, a non-digestible part of plant cells, is considered significant toward reduction of the risk of certain types of cancer, particularly colon and rectal cancers as well as the lowering of blood cholesterol. Fiber adds bulk to the diet and speeds up the passage of food through the digestive system, shortening the time that cancer-causing agents from food would remain in the body.

Top sources of fiber include dried legumes (beans, peas, and lentils), prunes, figs, apricots, whole-grains, mangoes, pears, apples, Brussels sprouts, seeds, nuts, berries, citrus fruits, potatoes and cruciferous vegetables.

[The Conscious Rasta's recommended daily allowance for fiber should be over 50 grams a day. Remember, in East Africa they average 70+ grams and they have very low incidence of heart disease and no colorectal disease!]

Cruciferous vegetables (broccoli, cauliflower, Brussels sprouts, kohlrabi and cabbage), as well as carrots and onions, contain sulforaphane which activates enzymes that protect against cancer.

The most healthful foods can lose their nutritional value before they ever reach your plate because certain vitamins and minerals can be lost or destroyed during cooking. To reduce the nutrient loss of foods you can use acids such as lemon juice, other citrus juices, or vinegar to slow enzyme activity in fruits and vegetables which can lead to the destruction of beta carotene, vitamin C, E, and other vitamins. In addition, refrigerating or freezing foods slows destructive enzyme activity. Further, the longer foods are stored or cooked, the more vitamins they generally lose.

Chapter 8 – Food Wars for the 21ˢᵗ Century

The Population Control Conspiracy

Long-term followers of the Conscious Rasta Perspective know of my persistent concern over what my research indicates as a global population control agenda intended to severely regulate the numbers of fast-growing populations around the globe. According to reams of data that I've collected over the past few years, those most at risk of being caught up in this massive culling of humankind are Blacks throughout Africa, the Caribbean and within designated "Third World" urban centers in industrialized nations, along with southern Asians and large numbers of Latin Americans in the Western hemisphere.

I have often cited U.S. government national security-related documents such as:

- Henry Kissinger's population study entitled **U.S. National Security Study Memorandum 200: "The Implications of Worldwide Population Growth on U.S. Security and Overseas Interests" (NSSM200)** which specifically identified 15 countries for which strategies would be developed to counter their rapid population growth. Those nations are Nigeria, Ethiopia, Egypt, Indonesia, Pakistan, Brazil, the Philippines, Bangladesh, Mexico, Columbia, India, Turkey and Thailand.

- Zbigniew Brzezinski's **Global 2000 Report to the President** which assessed the impact of projected population growth between 1975 and 2000 on the world's resources, environment and food sustenance and suggested that the planet would be much better off if the global population were reduced to figures closer to those of the early 1940s.

- Department of Defense (DOD) reports, such as one prepared for the U.S. Army in 1991 entitled **"Population Change and National Security"** which noted that rapid population growth in the developing world was likely to "create an international environment even more menacing to the security prospects of the Western alliance than was the Cold War for the past generation."

- The growth of an interlocking network of government and non-government agencies and organizations involved in population control activities which included such entities as: the CIA, DOD, US Agency for International Development, Centers for Disease Control and Prevention, the Council on Foreign Relations, various organs of the United Nations (World Health Organization, World Bank, UNICEF, UN Fund for Population Activities, etc.), Planned Parenthood International, International Committee of the Red Cross, Doctors Without Borders, the Club of Rome, Rockefeller and Ford Foundations, International Monetary Fund, private lobbies such as Zero Population Growth and Negative Population Growth, World Resources Council along with a host of greater and lesser neo-Malthusian advocates around the globe.

The second edition of these Conscious Rasta Reports, **_POPULATION WAR: Report from the Frontline_**, detailed the existence of this global network and illustrated much of the rapid demographic shift which has set this 'genocide society' upon its killing/sterilizing mission.

Food as a Weapon of War

I have collected a number of important documents that have led me to conclude that over the course of the coming decades, food deprivation will increasingly be used as a tool by which large groups of targeted populations will find survival more difficult. Certain trends going back to the mid-1980s demonstrate that the spread of famine within certain geographic regions can be linked to security policies of food exporters like the United States and that deliberate strategies caused these destructive famines.

In addition, influential organizations such as the Council on Foreign Relations and Worldwatch Institute have prophesied widespread famine and food deprivation for the foreseeable future, specifically identifying Sub-Saharan Africa and southern Asia as most likely affected by food shortages.

The brevity of portions of this report are not indicative of the seriousness which should be attached to the threat of widespread "food wars" in the future. The data which I have collected to confirm this concept is extensive. My interpretation of that data, disseminated through dozens of previously published research reports (a few in excess of 200 pages), motivates me to continue to deposit volumes of ink to depict this concept of widespread food deprivation as a tactical weapon in a global "clash of civilizations" between that part of humankind lovingly referred to as "The West" and segments of the same human family denigrated as the "Third World." Not only does the data exist to illustrate how this clash is brewing but those conducting the assault have produced an even greater mass of propaganda rationalizing the need to commit such an assault.

The Rise and Fall of the Green Revolution

In the immediate decades following Europe's World War II, there occurred throughout the globe an explosion of agricultural productivity which significantly increased the daily caloric intake of persons in lesser-developed countries (LDCs). This success of the Green Revolution has largely been attributed to industrialized farming methods which used technology and chemistry to turn large areas which had not yet been developed for agriculture into productive land. Yet those same high-tech methods which relied upon agricultural machinery and chemicals often created conditions which quickly depleted the once-virgin soil of its basic nutrients, causing topsoil erosion, accelerated desertification (the slow encroachment of deserts on fertile regions) and destruction of forests which were an important component of the natural environment.

The Green Revolution persisted throughout the 1960s, began to wane during the latter part of the 1970s and reversed itself by the mid-1980s. In the developing world, food production rose by an average of 117% in the quarter of a century between 1965 and 1990. Grain production grew annually by 29 million tons between 1950 and 1990, an overall increase of 169% despite an increase in land-under-production of only 17%. Fish catch increased from 9 to 19 kilograms per capita. Record human population increase during the same period was attributed to this widespread availability of foodstuffs as well as the introduction of widespread sanitation and water-delivery systems.

For Africa, benefits of the Green Revolution began to peter out during the early 1970s. Before that period, between the period of independence, commencing with Ghana in 1957 and the downturn in growth of gross domestic product (GDP) in the early 1970s, certain African countries, such as Nigeria, Ghana and Kenya, had been on growth curves which rivaled or exceeded such modern economic successes as Korea, Taiwan and Malaysia. Other African countries, namely Angola, Zaire, South Africa, Senegal and Uganda among others, had equal potential to develop into economic and development powerhouses as soon as they would be able to cast off the shackles which colonial powers still held over them. But African nations' conditions began to rapidly sour and the downward spiral has seemed to continue unabated. The main reason for the inability of Africa to sustain its economic development was due to the post-colonial dependence on former colonial masters which African leaders could not, or would not shake. Nearly all of those countries who did achieve true independence somehow succumbed to tribal rivalry and catastrophic civil warfare. Tanzania seems to be the notable exception.

Dependent upon external superpowers, many nations imported food stocks which, before the colonization period, they had previously produced for self. The largest grain-producers severely cut production and scaled back exports in the mid-1980s. In the U.S., grain production, which had climbed to as high as 140 million tons annually, with nearly half of that entering foreign markets, was reduced during the Reagan administration to nearly half. Farmers are now subsidized to keep land out of production. Subsequently, exports to grain-importing nations became more costly and donations to hungry populations became increasingly nonexistent.

Such policies contributed directly to the first of the modern geopolitical famines, that which affected Ethiopia in 1984. The Ethiopian catastrophe resulted from a combination of: a) superpower rivalry between the capitalist West (led by the United States) and the Marxist East (led by the Soviet Union) over the strategic Horn of Africa with its back-door access to the heart of the oil-producing regions; b) political conflicts and tribal rivalries within Ethiopia which crushed farmers and misappropriated their lands; c) a breakdown in infrastructure by which excess foodstuffs would be transported between regions; and d) the targeting of Ethiopia within U.S. national security policy as one of 13 countries whose population growth would pose strategic competition in the coming decades unless that trend were reversed.

Malthusian Projections of Mass Starvation

Modern-day proponents of the (largely discredited) theories of the 18th century English economist Thomas Parsons Malthus, have claimed for decades that rapid population growth around the world will eventually outstrip food production unless effort is made to check population-increase. They are quick to point to the conditions of such countries as Ethiopia, Somalia, Bangladesh and other lesser-developed regions and claim that the rapidly-breeding peoples of those regions have exhausted their capacity to feed themselves and thus are dooming their entire region to catastrophe if they don't get with the "family planning" program.

Neo-Malthusians have reserved a special contempt for Sub-Saharan Africa. Perhaps the most insidious piece of anti-African propaganda I have ever encountered appeared in the so-called "liberal" journal The Nation, May 27, 1996, authored by Christopher Hitchens. In his article entitled "Africa Adrift", Hitchens drew upon some of the most contemptible analogies to the continent's present condition imaginable, all this in an article seemingly critical of the Neo's. I will only repeat the worst of various metaphors used in the article, which Hitchens excepted from a book written by Conor Cruise O'Brien, **On the Eve of the Millennium**. That extraction itself was annexed from the German political theorist Friedrich Nietzsche:

> The hands of survivors cling to the sides of the boat.
> But the boat has already as many passengers as it
> can carry.   No   more   survivors   can   be

accommodated, and if they gather and cling on, the boat will sink, and all be drowned. The captain orders out the hatchets. The hands of the survivors are severed. The lifeboat and its passengers are saved.

Throughout the media, blaring headlines are replete with scalding condemnations of the plight of struggling populations, particularly those in Africa. Such headlines as "Africa: the Scramble for Existence", "A New Colonialism: Europe Must Go Back Into Africa" and "Colonialism's Back – and Not a Moment Too Soon" scream vulgar epithets at the whole continent and create in the subconscious mind of the unsympathetic reader a disassociation, perhaps the acceptance of the probability of wholesale abandonment, or worse yet the idea of actually putting Africans out of their wretched misery. In the American John Wayne tradition, isn't it better to die quickly from a bullet to the brain than to lie starving in the dust while vultures and hyenas wait impatiently in the shadows for the chance to steal the flesh from your still-breathing carcass?

Important Trends for the Future

Famine

Since the late 1970s, a nearly-continuous series of famines has devastated countries like Bangladesh, Ethiopia, Somalia, Mozambique, Liberia, India, Sudan, and Angola smaller regions surrounding the Sahara Desert. These could likely be the result of population-reduction strategies developed by the U.S. and its western allies. In other words, some of these famines could not have occurred, even amid severe drought, if other social and political factors had not contributed to a serious breakdown in food delivery systems.

Declining Grain Production

Significant reductions in grain production by food-producing nations, like the United States, have resulted from political policies intended to decrease excess grain stocks' exportation to dependent countries. In the case of the U.S. reduction in grain production, it was instigated despite subsequent negative economic impact due to diminished export revenue along with the need to subsidize farmers asked to keep land out of production. As well, it has resulted in spiraling food inflation within the very populations whose taxes support non-production. Due to such strategies, world grain stocks are at their lowest level in two decades, between 14% and 15% of annual consumption.

Post-Colonial Policies

An examination of colonial history from the 1800s to date yields an understanding of colonial-era and post-colonial-era policies that created dependence in former food-producing regions, in particular Africa. Walter Rodney's excellent book on the subject, **HOW EUROPE UNDERDEVELOPED AFRICA**, illustrated how European colonizers forced indigenous populations to curb subsistence crops' production cultivate cash crops desired by the colonial master, initially in order to pay hut taxes. Eventually this expanded to colony-wide production of agricultural products which were often of little use to the producing population, which would then be exported to Europe and America. The producing nations would be compensated little, if at all, for their commodity and the meager earnings would then be spent on food and other commodities produced in the foreign lands. Increasingly dependent on external supplies, nations were sold foodstuffs which were frequently undesired, spoiled, depleted of nutrients or otherwise incompatible to the dietary requirements of forced-consumers. The modern-day version of the colonial policy, food aid, has prolonged the same external dependence and increasingly, rich nations are severely cutting back aid to LDCs.

Structural Adjustment Policies

Largely through institutions like the World Bank and the International Monetary Fund, as well as direct-lending by other non-governmental organizations (NGOs), lending policies favoring the wealthy nations have decimated infrastructure within nations that have always had great potential for food self-sufficiency. Structural Adjustment Policies (SAPs) are part of a four-step policy which the West has developed to usurp upward mobility among LDCs. That four-step process, in brief goes as such: a) convince the target nation to significantly increase its production for export and to accept imported commodities and technology from foreign entities, b) encourage the exporter to increase exports through foreign financing, sowing the seeds for future debt-crisis, c) trigger the debt-crisis through devaluation of the exporter's commodity and currency on the world market (a "world" market controlled by the West), followed by a demand for radical changes in domestic policies and social priorities such as cutting back on government employees and scaling down infrastructure development – the dreaded SAP, and d) blame the increasing economic catastrophe on too-rapid population growth therefore requiring that further financial assistance will be tied to implementation of family planning measures (population control). SAPs suck the vitality out of a developing nation's economy. Policies of the major lending organizations too often reflect not the needs of the receiving nations but political expediencies for the rich benefactors. Thus the reason that India was the top recipient of World Bank loans in 1995 was not so much a matter of the critical motivation of poverty, but that India's former colonial headquarters, London, persuaded the bank to pursue a particular lending policy favoring its market interests. Japan has been a similar advocate for China, who has some $70 billion in foreign reserves. China and India are the two largest recipients of World Bank loans.

Low-Intensity Conflict

Internecine wars within certain regions have served to perpetuate conditions which lead to widespread famine. During the 40 year Cold War era, which was in essence a European conflict, proxy wars between the Western and Eastern European blocs materialized in distant places like Korea, Vietnam, Chile, Guatemala, the Congo (now Zaire), Angola, South Africa, Mozambique, Afghanistan, Ethiopia, Somalia, El Salvador, Nicaragua, Jamaica, Grenada, Ghana and numerous other locales where leaders had often, but not always, aligned with capitalist or Marxist camps. Today that process continues despite the demise of socialism. The latest alignment in the ever-shifting world of global conflicts is between the West (who always seem to be involved in worldwide ideological conflict) and the Islamic world. This "clash of civilizations" is currently involving Somalia, Palestine/Israel, the Persian Gulf states, Sudan, Libya, Nigeria, Algeria, Egypt and, to a lesser degree, within the United States. According to Samuel P. Huntington's landmark article "The Clash of Civilizations?" which appeared in Foreign Affairs, Summer 1993, "the conflicts of the future will occur along the cultural fault lines separating civilizations." Huntington makes two notable predictions in this significant article: a) the West's major adversary for the foreseeable future is that block of nations who identify with Islamic culture, and b) African civilization is on the verge of becoming nonexistent if certain destructive trends continue unabated.

Excesses of the Wealthy Nations

Greedy and selfish industrialized nations, led by the United States, have evolved along avenues which foment political and social conditions that waste food, subsidize non-production and lead to environmental destruction of shared world food stocks such as fishing reserves. An example of this devastation is the 50% decline in the annual salmon catch on the West Coast between 1985 and 1995 — from 42 tons down to 20.7 tons — largely due to U.S. environmental policies which have damaged once-pristine rivers in the Northwest. Within wealthy countries, and increasing in LDCs emulating Western values, bourgeois class desires for material consumption combine with expanding urban encroachment on farmland to further the conflict between that which is desired and that which is practical. Population-dense countries such as Britain, Belgium, Hong Kong, Japan, Taiwan, Korea and Germany, many of whom have scant natural resources, are having devastating impact on places like the tropical rain forests of Cameroon, the Philippines and Brazil, are depleting oceanic stocks off the coasts of Central and South America, Africa and southeast Asia, are exporting millions of tons of nuclear waste, toxic chemicals and agricultural pollutants, and are corrupting the social environment within poorer countries in pursuit of vampire-like "free trade" policies. All of these policies make sustainable production of foodstuffs increasingly more difficult. The irony is that many of these same destructive policies also undermine the ability of the offending nations to maintain their positions of power and influence – the rise of infertility in industrialized nations is a prime example of them cutting off their own testicles in their own greedy rush for materialism. Among the main culprits for destructive excess, the U.S. has seen its ranking among nations for low infant mortality fall from 3rd in the world in the late 1930s to 24th in 1995, ranking for life expectancy among selected developed countries shift from 7th in 1950 to 17th in 1990, and according to a June 1996 UNICEF report, attain the worst ranking among the richest nations, by far, for children living in poverty (compare for example the U.S. rate for child poverty—21% to France—6.5%) – a dismal record for "the greatest nation in the world."

Climatic Change

Apparent changes in weather patterns attributed to so-called global warming, natural disasters and rising epidemics of crop diseases have resulted in destroyed harvests, droughts, increased desertification, crop destruction and other conditions which have impaired food production and fomented conditions for rapid food inflation. These weather changes might range from extended cold-waves or heat-waves, early or late frost, record low or high-temperature seasons, years of substandard levels of rainfall, widespread flooding, record snowfalls, blizzards, tornadoes, hurricanes and ill-timed seasonal changes – all of which have the potential to interrupt the critical timing which agriculture must rely upon to deliver the predictable harvests required to feed sprawling nations. Crop diseases with such exotic names as whirling disease among Rocky Mountain trout fisheries, Karnal blunt fungus, which has caused the destruction of thousands of acres of wheat in California, Arizona, New Mexico and Texas "potentially endangering America's entire $4.9-billion wheat export program for this year and beyond", and duck-killing botulism outbreaks in Riverside and Long Beach, California – these are but three examples of such disease outbreaks which could seriously impact international food supplies in the coming decades. Periodic insect invasions of cockroaches, locusts and grasshoppers still cause widespread crop destruction around the globe, often provoking mass pesticide spraying which itself is long-term destructive.

The Cancerous Practices of Agribusiness

High-technology farm industrialization which relies heavily upon an ever-expanding array of chemical pesticides, herbicides and fertilizers has resulted in widespread contamination of formerly reliable food and water sources. Adding to that, manufacturers in the U.S. produce some 6.7 trillion pounds of chemicals each year, more than 26,000 pounds for every man, woman and child, much of which is banned for use in this country and exported to countries where the tainted substances are allowed. In many instances, the embargoed chemicals, which include DDT and DES, make their way quickly back into the U.S. food chain through imported food stocks, fruits and vegetables out of season, grown in countries whose lax environmental laws allow the use of chemicals prohibited in this country. Large-scale farming, which has virtually destroyed the tradition of the 'family farm', has fomented massive soil erosion, ground water contamination, proliferation of chemicals which have profound endocrine-disrupting consequences and contaminating farm workers, along with the consuming public, with hundreds of substances for which the long-term negative side effects have never been determined. Because of the power and influence of a massive agribusiness political lobby, policies such as the phase-out of the nasty pesticide methyl bromide in California which was scheduled to have occurred in June 1996 has been delayed to January 2001. The consequences of this political decision, which involved California Governor Pete Wilson and his allies in the agribusiness industry, could have deadly results for countless farmworkers, at least 18 of whose deaths have been attributed to methyl bromide.

International Market Agreements

Dubious "Free Trade" treaties such as NAFTA and GATT have the potential to create massive environmental destruction within developing countries. Rainforest depletion, nuclear dumping, chemical exportation, and sub-minimum wage slave-like working conditions can be expected to produce circumstances adverse to small-scale agriculture within weaker nations. This will likely also contribute to demands for export crop and undermine time-honored traditions of subsistence farming. Many well-informed observers have warned that this signals the development of an Earth, Inc. to be managed by all-powerful multinational corporations whose attitude signals that costs-verses-risk will jeopardize the health and self-interests of peasant workers to the advantage of the corporate bottom line. This fuels the development of a big corporation attitude of "Eat the poor – it's good for profits!"

Rich Nations' "Third-World" Sub-Populations

economic and social policies of wealthy countries isolate and impoverish vulnerable ethnic and social groups within their own borders, creating conditions ripe for malnutrition. A tragic example is that of the so-called African-American, who after 400 years of coexistence with his former enslavers, still cannot seem to achieve a semblance of socio-economic equality and political justice. Thus, nearly complete dependence upon this historic oppressor for the basic sustenance's of life – food, clothing and shelter – puts Blacks, along with other vulnerable groups (to include poor Whites) in an undesirable position on the eve of the 21st century. By every measure, America is extremely hostile to its poor. The gross disparity between rich and poor, high numbers of children trapped in poverty, and spiraling costs of basic sustenance all forecast a dangerous future for such populations as we enter a time when anxieties over population control, rising unemployment, the implosion of the social security net and racial tensions are rising. For a sub-population to then be totally reliant upon selfish corporations for food, and significant numbers of the minority to be dependent on welfare is an extremely perilous position to be caught in.

Anti-People Propaganda

Throughout the media we can now identify a proliferation of propaganda aimed at establishing the mindset by which certain "Third World" populations within industrialized nations are being set up for a reduction of numbers. A follow-through with this analysis leads one to determine that the targets of such 'hate rhetoric' will be likely eventually be abandoned and allowed to starve. What does a nation such as the U.S., suffering from declining productivity, rising ethnic conflict, diminishing world economic status and increasing fears of a strife-driven future – what does such a country (with the genocidal history of America) do with an undesired population? What becomes of "redundant labor", "useless eaters" and "a poor and defiant black population...confined to urban ghettos indefinitely into the future"? If you are in the dominant class's position, do you continue to feed them despite their unwillingness toward productivity and anti-social attitudes? If America truly has had a long-standing "Negro problem" why should this country go out of its way to continue feeding such a population?

Ill-Conceived Policies of Developing Populations

Undoubtedly, with proper foresight, planning, regenerative food-production methods and a commitment to farming research and infrastructure development, those groups at greatest risk of being injured by food wars (predominantly Africa, southeast Asia, parts of Latin America and "Third World" populations within urban centers of the industrialized countries) could've long ago reversed the conditions which made them vulnerable to such attack. In most cases political leadership has either lacked the will, vision or independence-of-action with regard to implementing a self-serving agenda and to force their constituency to make required changes before the greatest period of suffering occurs. Increasing we are determining that such ineffective (but persisting) leadership has unsavory connections to the forces of control through covertly-administered networks for obedience. Thus, groups who seem to be always searching for a proverbial 'messiah' to lead them, find themselves, generation after generation, on the short end of divine promises unmet and heavenly ambitions unfulfilled. The saintly old songs of "We Shall Overcome", "Oh Happy Day" and "Amazing Grace" will do little to fill the bellies of hungry babies in the brutal reality of the New World Order. An aggressive new style of leadership based upon correct analysis, non-emotionalism, deliberation and strategic planning must come to the fore to fend off the massive culling of the coming food wars and population wars.

Conclusion to Food Wars

According to my own calculations, there is an increasingly narrow window during which we can interrupt this continued decline in our political and social condition which serves to fulfill neo-Malthusian prophesies of mass starvation. On the micro level, I do all that I can to urge individuals to take up vegetable gardening, shopping at farmers' markets and purchasing in cooperative networks, thereby learning the methods of small-scale food production and distribution. On the level beyond that I try to point out that the abandonment of rural lands for the lure of metropolitan centers has put certain populations, such as my own, in dire predicament. African people, the progenitors of the science of agriculture on the planet are now increasingly stigmatized as being incapable of feeding themselves.

The African continent, with its immense size, mineral wealth, abundance of water, forests, animals and fertile soils, has been largely colonized and socialized into a state of food-dependence upon external suppliers. African-Americans, along with Africans throughout the Diaspora, have overwhelmingly turned their backs on the plight of their homeland, the only place which will unselfishly extend them refuge when the West can no longer tolerate their presence in the lands which it has appropriated for its own diminishing numbers of children.

What will it take to motivate the myriad sons and daughters of Africa, along with genuinely sympathetic populations in equally-despised southern Asia and Latin America, to stand up, take the reins of history firmly in our own rugged hands, and reconnect ourselves directly with the self-reliant principles which have so lovingly embraced us from the dawn of our existence on this plane? My brothers and sisters, what is it going to be? How can we expect to survive if we produce no food with which to nourish our precious babies?

References for Food Wars of the 21st Century

1)   ENVIRONMENT GROUP PREDICTS FOOD SHORTAGE from the Associated Press, Long Beach Press Telegram 1994

2)   CAN THE GROWING HUMAN POPULATION FEED ITSELF? by John Bongaarts, Scientific American, March 1994

3)   FACING FOOD INSECURITY by Lester R. Brown, and CARRYING CAPACITY: EARTH'S BOTTOM LINE by Sandra Postel, from State of the World 1994, WorldWatch Institute, 1994

4)   RICE BOWLS AND DUST BOWLS by Robert L. Paarlberg, Foreign Affairs Vol. 75, No. 3, May/June 1996

5)   THE CLASH OF CIVILIZATIONS? by Samuel P. Huntington, Foreign Affairs, Vol. 72, No. 3, Summer 1993

6)   TROUBLED WATERS: HARD TIMES SURFACE IN BRITISH COLUMBIA SALMON INDUSTRY by Craig Turner, Los Angeles Times, June 13, 1996

7)   WORLD BANK LOSES ITS WAY, an editorial appearing in the Los Angeles Times, February 13, 1996

8)   CLINTON PLAN CALLS FOR REMOVING 2 DAMS TO RESTORE SALMON RUNS by Kim Murphy, Los Angeles Times, March 20, 1996

9)   ILLNESS PUTS TROUT-FISHING INDUSTRY IN HOT WATER by Louis Sahagun, Los Angeles Times, June 1996

10)   WHEAT INFECTION FOUND IN STATE; BLYTH AREA QUARANTINED by Chris Kraul, Los Angeles Times, March 30, 1996

11)   SEEDS OF DESTRUCTION: SPREAD OF FUNGUS POSES THREAT TO U.S. WHEAT HARVEST by Chris Kraul, Los Angeles Times, April 3, 1996

12)   BOTULISM KILLS DUCKS IN RIVERSIDE by Phil Pitchford, Long Beach Press Telegram, October 20, 1995

13)   SNOWS UNSETTLE PRODUCE PRICES IN SOUTHLAND by Kenneth Chang, Los Angeles Times, January 13, 1996

14)   U.S. CHILD POVERTY WORST AMONG RICHEST NATIONS by Robin Wright, Los Angeles Times, June 12, 1996

15)   EARTHWATCH: A DIARY OF THE PLANET – INSECT INVASION from the Los Angeles Times, May 2, 1996

16)   WINDS OF CHANGE from Foreign Affairs, Fall 1990

17)   MINORITY REPORT: AFRICA ADRIFT by Christopher Hitchens, The Nation, May 27, 1996

18)   AFRICA: THE SCRAMBLE FOR EXISTENCE by Lance Murrow, Time, September 7, 1992

19)   A NEW COLONIALISM: EUROPE MUST GO BACK INTO AFRICA by William Pfaff, Foreign Affairs, January/February 1995

20)   COLONIALISM'S BACK – AND NOT A MOMENT TOO SOON by Paul Johnson, New York Times Magazine, April 18, 1993

Chapter 9 – Organic Gardening

It's 1992 in America. Corporate monopolies have taken over political systems, the military establishment, absconded with the nation's economic potential, and usurped the energy, healthcare and food producing systems within this nation and others.

Widespread famine, cancer, heart disease, birth defects, immune disorders, violence, food, drug, and alcohol addiction have become raging epidemics in the global community. Against all modern trends the average lifespan for African-Americans is stagnant.

How much longer can you trust these corporations to supply you and your children with the basic sustenance of life that is food? – Keidi Awadu

When I wrote that as introduction to my book **The Organic Gardener**, I anticipated that the system by which most of us obtain our food was in bad shape and getting worse each year. Four years later, the trend continues and even worse, looming on the horizon of the 21st century are food wars as part of continuing "clashes of civilizations."

Today the food and water supply systems are disastrously compromised because of several factors including:

- agricultural chemicals, pesticides & herbicides

- heavy metal pollutants, food additives and complex molecules

- waterborne parasites & toxic chemicals

- mind control drugs and social engineering

- top prices being charged for poor quality products

- food inflation

- age-old survival skills are withering away

- stress, lack of exercise, toxic overload, etc., resulting from disconnection from nature

- crises triggered by climatic conditions and global warming

- population control and eugenics protocols targeting food-dependent countries

Yet there is a relatively simple solution to get out of this dependence -- small-scale, labor-intensive organic vegetable gardening. Consider this:

1) Land exists, just look around your own home or share space with family or friends.

2) You probably already have the extra time; you're just wasting it with nonproductive activities.

3) Consider the payoff of this investment: ten to twelve hours a week for family of four combined with an automatic watering system and other supplies which amount to about $500 initial investment should be expected to produce approximately $75 worth of

organic food   each week, from a relatively small backyard plot.

4) Be expected to notice dramatic health improvement from organic gardening including weight loss and chronic disease prevention.

5) Food production is a commonsense engagement requiring self-education, and self-empowerment.

6) Project this knowledge and capability forward into the future through your children.

7) Make your historic oppressor's best laid plans backfire by becoming independent.

There is a whole new world of food independence waiting, like an untapped gold mine, in your own back yard. Exploit it!

I want to welcome as many of you as possible to the joys and benefits of organic gardening. I hope to prove that you, like I, can develop a productive, pesticide free source of fruits and vegetables in as small a space as an average urban backyard, even a condo balcony. In as few as thirty days you can be enjoying fresh organic food. In sixty days, you can have enough harvest to freeze, can, share with good friends (better friends, now) and still have fresh food daily.

In addition, for me the garden is always welcoming. Though I get so busy on certain days that I'm frantic, it is always a captivating pleasure to enter the garden and be surrounded by vital life-force, fresh scents and greenery.

There are commercial organic gardens throughout the country, and many are available for brief tours. Most cities provide community gardening space that can be rented for a small yearly fee. Therefore, the family living in a condo or apartment can realize some of the benefits that the homeowner might readily utilize.

A garden greenhouse, constructed from inexpensive materials, could provide uninterrupted growth through the worst of winter in most southern states and is a good way of defending one's organic interests from unwanted pollution or pesticide spraying.

Getting Started

The basics of gardening begin at soil preparation and this phase of gardening is absolutely critical to both the amount of crops which will be produced and the ease with which production occurs. It is feasible to start germinating seeds indoors or in starter sets while you prepare your beds. This will give you a head start on your harvest date.

For germinating seeds you can obtain reusable starter pots at any nursery, peat pots filled with organic potting mix or even a margarine dish, with a few holes in the bottom, filled with inexpensive vermiculite and placed in a plate of fresh water.

If you have not previously grown on your plot or are digging up turf to create the space then careful preparation of your soil will alleviate headaches later. Several fundamental concerns must be dealt with.

A good first step is to determine if your soil is too acidic or alkaline. Soil that is not within the proper pH range will develop stunted and underdeveloped plants that, no matter how you fertilize them, will not bear fruit properly.

A pH test kit is available at your local nursery or from county agricultural agencies. Ideal range is a pH of 6.5 to 7. You may need to add lime (too acid) or sulfur (too alkaline) to correct it. This step may mean the difference between a bountiful harvest or months of frustration.

If you are removing turf then it is absolutely essential that you get the deep roots out of your gardening plot otherwise grass will keep coming back and aggressively compete with your vegetables for nutrients. You want no competition from grass or weeds. The proper tool for this job is a digging fork as it will reach down more than ten inches to rip up the deepest roots. Repeat cleaning of a previously sodden area for about four days and you will avoid a lot of problems with grass.

Soil texture is extremely important and nearly all soil needs amendment. Sandy soil will not hold water. Clay soil causes water runoff and summer heat will harden it like concrete. Ideal soil is rich with humus, which is decaying vegetable matter, and holds water well yet drains quickly. You should add a four-inch layer of soil amend, composted nitro humus, gromulch, peat moss, other organic compost or such soil enhancements as perlite and vermiculite, which are puffed silicates that hold moisture in the soil. You then blend in the soil amendments to a minimum of ten inches deep. Correctly blended soil is free of weeds, rocks and you can thrust your hand into it easily up to the wrist. At this point you must concern yourself with making the healthiest environment for plant roots. Do not walk on your prepared beds.

Some vegetables are better when started as seeds but a trip to the nursery for seedlings can give several weeks jump on harvest day. Transplanting is an art. Proper soil texture, careful handling of delicate root balls and the correct amount of watering are the keys to healthy transplants.

When planting or transplanting you should add a small amount of fertilizer to facilitate good root growth. As we are concerned with organic gardening, free from pesticides and chemicals, seriously consider which fertilizers you use. Organic types such as manure, blood or bone meal and fish emulsion are natural, biodegradable, and non-toxic byproducts as opposed to petroleum-based chemicals. A balance such as 5-10-10 is ideal for seedlings and this type of fertilizer makes for healthy roots.

Garden Organization, Layout, and Design

By planning for the space available you will hopefully avoid problems created by too little or too much sun, sprawling plants, pests, insufficient or excessive yield as well as losing food to predators, human and animal. Does your space include sunny walls? Which side is best for which crop, North, South, East, or West? Is there trash or clutter close to your garden? How much space is necessary for your family size?

These questions should figure well in your garden plan. North and East facing walls will be cooler and less sunny than South or West sides. You can use walls for vertical growing and vining plants, tomatoes, beans, cucumbers and melons will be perfectly suited. Proper placement of plants increases yield substantially, provides additional control for weeds and pests, means easy maintenance and makes the garden look good.

Vertical growing requires some sort of support frame. This can be as simple as 5 foot poles stuck in the ground, twine tied to some sort of bracket, or a large meshed sturdy fence supported by posts. For heavier fruits sturdiness is a must. Melons can be tied to a strong fence with wide strips of cloth functioning as bras. The wide mesh allows for reaching through the fence for house maintenance, pulling weeds or harvesting.

Squash, cucumbers, and melons grown horizontally require lots of space. Read carefully the spacing on the back of your seed packs. Usually they can be planted closer than the instructions state but this style of "square foot" gardening requires careful attention. Be aware of the productivity of your crop as the ground space required for a horizontal harvest of melons might provide weeks' worth of something else. Tomatoes, such hardy producers, can overwhelm you with their harvest. Only three to six feet of a wall should be dedicated to each type of these heavy producers.

Key to success in planning your garden layout is interplanting your vegetables in a manner so that they will maximize the available space. In addition, correct placement will facilitate ease of care and in certain instances thwart pests.

Certain vegetables such as radishes, lettuce and spinach grown quite rapidly compared to other slow growers like Brussels sprouts, corn, melons, or eggplant. If you are forced to garden in limited space, then it can be quite useful to interplant so that as one crop matures and is harvested the adjacent crop is ready to take over the vacated space.

Radishes are an example of a crop which can be planted between any other seeds. During late spring, this vegetable can be ready to harvest in thirty days. At that time, a second crop such as carrots might just be reaching a size that would have put it into competition with an adjacent plant.

The relative position of the sun as seasons change must be considered when placing vegetables in the garden. It can be self-defeating to plant corn, Brussels, tomatoes or another tall crop so that as they mature they cut the sun from short crops inadvertently placed behind them. I recommend placing certain tall or vining crops along walls that receive direct sun. If there is only a foot or two available along the wall, it is then possible to interplant short crops at the foot of the walled crop. Trellises, wide-mesh fencing, bamboo canes or poles can direct vining crops up high in the air as the remaining foot space is reserved for another.

Stages of Growth

Plants have various stages that each require a particular kind of attention. The first stage is the sprouting of the seed and establishment of a root system. During the first weeks of a plants growth it is particularly susceptible to pests that can shear off the entire plant at ground level overnight. An effective shield against nasty snails, slugs and cutworms can be made from used plastic milk containers. Simply cut the bottom off a milk jug, cut it at the top leaving at least a four-inch hole for circulation and leaving six or so inches of the sides. Make certain that the bottom ring is firm against the soil so that no pests can climb under the barrier.

After a few weeks of growth, when the plant has established roots and a fair amount of leaf growth, flowers begin to form on fruiting plants. Many plants are self-pollinating and develop two kinds of flowers. Male flowers are characterized by a long stem and generally appear before the shorter female flowers. Often a fruit will form from the female flower yet wither and die before reaching harvest size. This is usually because it was not pollinated. Having a healthy host of insects, called "beneficials" in the garden usually accomplishes the pollination without much help. Again, beneficials are a good reason to avoid pesticides.

I try to feed my garden every three weeks with various types of organic fertilizer. Container-grown plants may require feeding each two weeks because frequent watering strips nutrients from the soil, which is important in warm climates. Choice of organic fertilizers will vary; your experience will determine your favorites. My favorite is fish emulsion, a foul-smelling concoction that promotes rapid growth. Blood meal, bone meal, "compost tea," guano, manure, and other organic fertilizers also work well.

Composting

A vital key to organic gardening is to start a compost heap. Contrary to popular opinion, a compost heap should not stink. Properly prepared and maintained, a compost heap will be clean-smelling, easy to maintain, and after one to three months should yield nearly all your soil amendment and mulch needs, thereby saving you big bucks over the year.

The first step to a compost heap is a framed structure to build up the material. A reasonable construction might be of chicken wire reinforced with 2 by-4's or a frame made from discarded wooden skids. The main requirements will be: (1) a sturdy yet flexible frame, (2) an open side to insert organic materials, (3) the easy circulation of air, (4) the ability to turn the soil over with a digging or manure fork every week or so.

Materials that go in the compost heap should include:

- fallen leaves, spoiled fruits, and garden pruning

- grass clippings (unless from chemically treated turf)

- spent stems and roots (avoid weed seeds)

- kitchen scraps except for meat (meat scraps stink and attract dogs and cats)

- finely chopped tree limbs and stalks

- composted manure

- a few shovels of living soil to provide microorganisms

- earthworms and organic microorganism blends

Use fertilizers composed of a high percentage of free nitrogen to offer nutrients to the bacteria that transform compost into rich humus. Fertilize your heap at least once every couple of weeks and water it regularly. Treat it like a growing plant because you are growing the many tiny organisms that break down the organic matter into humus. With your sturdy digging fork, turn the compost heap ingredients once a week to keep air circulating throughout the lower layers and avoid foul odors. Composting is a simple, easy, and satisfying endeavor. Organic gardeners take no small measure of pride in their composting styles.

Planting for the Seasons

Cool Weather Planting

Much of my lifetime of gardening experience took place in California, which has three growing seasons: two cool and one warm. Planting for the cools seasons, which begin in January and September, and each lasts about four months, requires careful crop selection.

Seed selection during a cool season includes lettuce, leafy greens, radishes, beets, broccoli, cauliflower, carrots, onions, Brussels sprouts, cabbage, watercress, fancy greens, peas, potatoes, turnips, and countless herbs. Visit your local nursery or library and pick up a book in advance of the season so you can enjoy all your favorites. Many cool-season crops can be started indoors as seedlings so that the time outside can be extended weeks beyond tolerable weather conditions.

For strawberry fans, the cool season is a good time to plant a strawberry bed. Pick an area where the afternoon sun is relatively cool. Prepare your beds as previously advised, with deep loose soil rich with humus. It's good to border your strawberry bed with 1-by-8 boards so that you can raise the foundation above ground level. This will help to block access to slugs, snails, centipedes, and other crawling pests. Copper strips can also be nailed to raised-bed boards over which slugs and snails cannot crawl – the copper causes a chemical reaction that destroys the pests. When planting strawberries, use organic bone meal as fertilizer for good root growth. Commercially grown strawberries are among the most pesticide-laced fruits marketed. If you are as big a strawberry fan as me (at my Ohio childhood home, we grew seven 100-foot rows each spring), commercial contamination is all the more reason to grow your own!

If you cannot find a cool spot, you can purchase shade cloth from your local nursery or hardware supply. Use green or black netting to block the day's harshest sun so that newly planted tender plants won't dry out and die within the first weeks. This is also helpful for extending lettuce and tender greens into hotter weather where normally they would've gone to seed.

We frequently encounter unseasonable heatwaves in California. It may be an early or extended summer. I recall January weather in the mid-to-upper 90s and Septembers as well, which never really did cool down. This can require replanting succulent greens, peas, roots, and other cool-weather crops which don't fare well when it's too hot. Sometimes plants survive the heat but are stunted, withered, or rooted in crispy topsoil, resulting from not getting down to watering duties on those hot afternoons.

So, if you find yourself with stunted seedlings, don't delay replanting, transplanting, mulching down areas, and tilling close around tender seedlings. The key is to get them started growing again as soon as possible.

If there is a patch where spotted clumps of seedlings survived, then a suitable treatment might be as such:

- Locate a new patch to transplant (be sure to consider direct sun, vining, crowding, and accessibility) to maximize your space usage.

- Compost or amend the new spot, add bone meal or another organic high in phosphorus and potash and mix up the soil to 8 inches deep.

- Carefully spade 3 inches or more around the hardened base of surviving seedlings to 6 inches deep, lift the entire block of dirt out of the hole and place it in water.

- After the soil has partially loosened from the roots, place the seedling in the new bed with a gentle touch, be careful to set the root crown above ground level with a little mound.

- Pat a shallow bowl 6 inches around the new location.

- Hand water with a cup or watering bucket for the first week.

This re-transplant method should prove nearly 100% effective. Be alert to the presence of underground grubs and larvae when preparing a bed. These little thugs and bandits are often lurking, anxious to devour your seedling's tender roots.

Warm Weather Planting

During the months of May and June is the proper time to plant warm-season crops. These include hanging vegetables such as tomatoes, beans, eggplant, and cucumbers, other flowering crops like corn, all melons, and squashes. Particular attention must be paid to planting times as a plant will likely be stunted and unproductive if grown out of season. You don't want to waste the time or space.

The key here is to anticipate the seasonal change without planting too early or too late. Planting too early might produce wildly overgrown plants or vines, gangly structures with little or no flowers and vulnerability to pests that might not have been a problem if the timing had been correct. Planting too late requires fighting a broiling sun to get seedlings established or worse yet, growing tall strong plants that never get to flower and produce harvest because the weather changed again before the plant fully matured.

Careful attention to planting instructions which are included on the back of most seed packets will generally avoid the problem of planting out of season.

Water, Weeds, and Pests

Watering, weeds & pests will occupy much of your time with the garden. The organic garden will require careful attention because the "convenience" of toxic chemicals will not be available. This does not mean that you have to sacrifice your vegetables to weeds and bugs. Quite the contrary, organic gardening produces healthier plants which grow stronger and yield more, better tasting produce.

Watering in hot climates like our own in Southern California is a critical daily operation. Because of sandy soil, blistering midday heat and paucity of rainfall you will need a watering system that can overcome these obstacles so as to fully take advantage of the great growing seasons.

Sandy soil sheds it's water so quickly that without soil amendment you would need to water three times a day to keep the plants alive. By adding a few inches of quality mulch into the soil before planting you have created a soil that drains well yet holds water where the roots can get at it. An additional two inches of mulch, straw or dried grass clippings on the surface, surrounding your plants, will keep the water from evaporating too quickly. If you see your plants wilt it is the first sign that they need water quick.

Your garden should get a good watering everyday before 10:00 am. This timing works well in that there is nearly always enough moisture in the soil to get through the heat of the afternoon and has the added advantage of allowing the leaves and flowers to dry out before nightfall. Excess moisture on plants is a primary cause of leaf rot and other fungus diseases. Nighttime is when plants are most vulnerable so it's not recommended that you water the garden in the evening unless you absolute have to.

An automatic watering system is a wise investment. Consult your library or local building supply store for the proper manner to set up a sprinkler system. Also an automatic system can free up hours each month in maintenance time as well as to avoid mid-day burn during the worst heat of summer.

Weeds must be dealt with within the first few weeks of the season. After your plants have reached a certain size the weeds generally won't be able to compete. The best weed controls are a two inch layer of mulch and a careful eye.

Absolutely use no chemical weed killers anywhere in your garden. Space your plants so that you can easily access inner rows to maintain weed control.

Surely pests will migrate toward a healthy garden. It's a fact. You want to find a proper balance where they are not getting too much of your produce. Predator insects, also known as beneficials, feed on certain garden pests. Pesticides indiscriminately kill the beneficials with the unwanted bugs. Certain wasps, ladybugs, lacewings, and fungal bacteria available from your local nursery are good at controlling pests. Frequent inspection of your plants alerts you to the beginning of an infestation when control is much easier. A jet of water is quite effective at knocking pests off your plants. By battling the pests regularly, you interrupt their breeding cycle.   The organic garden requires daily attention mainly due to pests.

Caterpillar, slugs, cutworms, beetles, aphids, and the likes can be obnoxious. Yet you will maintain control if you are persistent. Never let the pests take over any part of your garden. Its a good practice to visit a library and study organic pest controls or two purchase a few books and magazines on the subject. It is, for the organic gardener, a never-ending educational experience learning to deal with various garden pests.

I have used various combinations of pest and fungus controls that are all non-toxic and sometimes unusual. They include:

1)   A solution of fiery hot peppers soaked for a couple of days in water then sprayed on leafy greens to deter aphids and leaf eaters.

2) Compost tea, which is made from soaking decaying material from the bottom of the compost heap in water in sunlight for a couple of days in order to transfer useful bacteria onto certain broad leaves, such as squash, peas, or melons. This prevents leaf fungus.

3) Bacillus thuringiensis (Bt), which is a common bacteria which kills leaf, corn and tomato-eating green worms.

4) Ladybugs and lacewings which are voracious consumers of aphids.

5) Insecticide soap, which is made from rendered animal fats, and causes soft-bodied pests to dry up in the sun by neutralizing their body oils.

6) Non-toxic copper solution to fight leaf and grape fungus.

7) Water jet to knock pests off the vegetables and interrupt their feeding/breeding cycle.

8) Hand-picking larger pests such as slugs, snails, beetles, grubs and grasshoppers and then immediately stomping them into the realm of their pest ancestors.

9) Setting out pie pans with a mixture of beer and snail bait (don't ever pug slug and snail bait directly on your soil – it is toxic!) into which the glutinous bastards crawl and drink themselves to death.

10) Using netting to protect fruit trees from birds, beetles and other flying pests.

11) Sticky pest resin, made from vegetable fats, to deter crawling pests such as slugs, ants, beetles, cutworms, mice or whatever – the resin can be applied to a paper tube collar or paper tape wrapped around the base of young trees or spread in a thin coat directly on the bark of mature trees.

12) Take small rubber balls, paint them as fully ripened fruit would look, screw in a hook, coat the fake fruit with pest resin and suspend it in the tree.

13) Hang sticky fly traps over the compost heap to decimate numbers of flies, whiteflies, wasps, gnats, mosquitoes, moths, beetles and others.

A Typical Daily Routine (About 1 Hour)

- Devote a particular time every day for gardening.

- First up is inspection. Look for pest damage, dry spots, ripe produce, and check to see that the plants are not growing over their boundaries.

- Tidy up the garden to maintaining its pleasant appearance. This goes a long way toward making the garden an enjoyable place to spend time.

- Bring out your plastic tub, brown paper bag, scissors or knife and harvest.

- After harvest spend a few minutes arranging vegetable beds, loosening up soil, pulling a few weeds, mulching down and, if necessary, cleaning out depleted beds and quickly replanting.

- When finished with harvesting, tidying and replanting it is time for the daily watering.

- Other frequent chores include turning the compost heap with a digging fork, pruning, trimming dead leaves, sweeping pathways, maintaining fences, etc.

- Allow at least 10 minutes or so just to meditate and enjoy the aura of the garden. A well-maintained garden is a joy to just stand in and soak up a little sun along with your plants.

- Try to include reading about gardening as part of your regular routine. It's possible to learn something every day about organic gardening.

Choosing Proper Garden Tools

As you spend more time with your garden you will inevitably find that your need for specialized tools becomes critical. Let us go over some of the most useful tools to be found in our gardens.

Most handy is the automated watering system or watering hose and attachments. The most convenient means of watering is by the use of an automated watering system or drip system. The cost is relatively modest and advantages great. For the person who must travel for more than a day or two without someone else water your garden, an automated watering system is a must. Check your local hardware store or garden nursery for a system and installation instructions.

For those who water by hand, a quality hose is a must. Cheap hoses will tangle, split, frustrate you and only last for a short season. A variety of attachments will be useful including: (1) an on-off valve attachment to control flow from the hose end, (2) 30" watering wand to put water where you want it and not drown the entire plant, (3) spray or gun attachment to wash down pests, dust and spider webs.   Other attachments can be useful for watering tree roots, (organic) liquid fertilizers, area watering or whatever your special needs.

Other necessary tools include:

1) a hand spade and fork for close-in work and transplanting

2) heavy tined digging fork for busting sod, removing deep roots, tossing the compost heap and working mulch deep into new beds

3) a leaf rake for adding leaves and mowed grass to the compost heap

4) a round-head shovel for digging and a square shovel for moving dirt and squaring beds

5) a tough rake for breaking up dirt clods, removing grass, weeds, sticks and stones

6) plastic tubs for moving dirt, carrying transplants, or harvesting

7) leather gloves

8) spray bottles for organic pesticides [remember, the organic gardener passionately avoids toxic chemicals]

9) a weeding rake (different from a lawn rake in that it is narrow and has usually only 4 tines)

10) plastic buckets for a variety of uses including recyclable kitchen scraps

11) a hand watering bucket for delicate transplants as well as mixing liquid fertilizers.

Surely there are many more tools than these. You will find that the above mentioned will suit most garden work.

Growing Culinary & Medicinal Herbs

With the experience of successful gardening season behind us, it is good to take on some fresh challenges for the garden. Adding an herb patch is something that you may imagine could be so pleasant. Try your hand at growing onions, parsley, peppers, rosemary, oregano, thyme, spearmint, peppermint, chives, watercress, sage, basil, anise, chamomile, lavender, cilantro, ganja and whatever herb seeds you can run across (I have grown all of the aforementioned).

Fresh herbs are generally easy to grow and provide the most heavenly fragrance imaginable. Fresh herbs make a perfect gift for close friends and family. Drying herbs for year-round use is also easy, economical, and practical.

The herbs you grow can be either culinary (for the kitchen) or medicinal, or both. As we are noting ever more oppressive government agencies bowing to pressure from pharmaceutical manufacturers and the medical-industrial complex, it is likely that we will one day be forced to grow our own medicinal herbs. The list of healing herbs is quite vast, and the key is obtaining seeds. There are excellent seed directories and alternative alliances throughout the world which provide healing herb seeds. Of course, with all the advantages of an organic, you will have much less need for radical healing anyway. Still it is pragmatic to take these necessary herbal remedies under our own power and control.

Aromatic herbs, such as lavender, sage, peppermint and lemon have shown potential as brain-hormone stimulants, increasing levels of serotonin in the brain. Serotonin is associated with feelings of fulfillment, calmness of mind and a good mood. Therefore, having a fresh sprig of herbs in a glass of water on your desk at work is a great way of creating an ambiance by which the work-a-day world is transformed into your own private oasis. Try it, it works!

From Garden to Storage

If you are as successful with your organic gardening endeavor as I have been, eventually you will need to answer one serious question: "What do I do with the excess harvest?

My gardening space is surprisingly limited, yet the amount of yield from this garden, developed to near maximum efficiency, is enough for six to ten people. While we do supplement our occasional dinner with store-bought consumables, or farmers' market-bought produce, there is usually no absolute need to do so.

My wife handles much of the chore of cleaning, freezing, and cooking. As she prepares the harvest, discarded leaves and stems enter a bucket which stands by the sink. Rinse water, spoiled fruits, and bug-chewed leaves all go into the bucket which then is recycled through the compost heap.

Excess produce cannot always be given away, so you can use a combination of freezing, canning, drying and other storage preparation which extends the useful life of fresh garden produce.

I do not have nearly enough space here to school anyone as to the myriad details of techniques in food storage. A trip to bookstore or health-food store may be necessary to peruse books and magazines on vegetable storage. Libraries are a wonderful community source for information. I periodically check out books on organic gardening, pest control, gardening techniques, freezing, canning, growing and drying herbs – obviously, there you can obtain books on a wide variety of subjects.

Leafy green vegetables, snap beans, carrots, peas and numerous other delicate to firm vegetables are easy to freeze. The trick is to heat the vegetables enough to stop natural enzyme and bacterial action without breaking down the cellular structure and turning the vegetables into mush. This is best accomplished by using a large cauldron of boiling water into which the vegetables are thrust for the briefest possible time (usually no more than 2 minutes), a metal strainer and a second large pot of iced water to stop the process. The entire operation from cleaning to freezer should take but ten minutes at the most.

Yet, when the freezer is full, canning is in order. This also is a good backup in case of extended power failure (perhaps an earthquake?). I searched around for a while looking for the familiar Ball ring jars before I finally discovered them above the pet food at the front of my local Lucky store. I suspect most chains should carry them but you'd be best to inquire by phone with the managers.

Canning tools include a deep cauldron or pressure cooker, food thermometer, tongs for handling hot jars and very careful attention to what you are doing. If you do not heat the food sufficiently, mold, bacteria or worse will destroy your efforts.   The jars form a vacuum seal which is indicated by an indentation of the jar lid, when successful.

Drying herbs is easier. Simply tie them on a string, wrap them once around with a piece of clean brown paper and hang them in a closet or garage free from dust and grit. Peppers can be dried in this manner also. Another great method for drying herbs is using a food dehydrator.

The Organic Gardening Spirit

People who tour my own garden are always in awe of the variety and quality of organic vegetables. It can be such a source of pride that I enjoy giving a running commentary of the characteristic of different plants.

What kind of people are organic gardeners?

Organic gardeners are difficult to pigeonhole. Certainly, many are vegetarians. That is an easy connection. For vegetarians a home-grown organic garden is paradise – a virtually cost-free source of food which is truly fit for gods.

Upwardly mobile people with an entrepreneur spirit make up a good portion of organic gardeners. It fits perfectly into economic as well as stress-busting regimens. You save at the grocery store at the same time you cut out the need for health club membership fees!

Cautious parents freely go the extra mile to assure their precious children have the best. Shouldn't this attitude extend itself to concern over pesticides, herbicides, chemical fertilizers, and food additives? You bet it should and just wait until you see your children eating fresh beans, corn and melons. Garden peas fresh from the pod beat sugary candy sweets any day in my house!

Gardening, specifically organic gardening, easily becomes a spiritual retreat. The combination of Earth, Sun, seed and sweat generates life-force and has profound effect on one's mood (serotonin levels?). I refer to it as my "grounding", wherein tensions caused by urban living get released as sweat and soil mixed.

There are times to just hang out in the garden, meditate and let time pass by as if it did not matter (ultimately, it doesn't). Sometimes you will find yourself behind schedule because the garden would not let you leave on time. Such pressure must not have really mattered so much in the first place.

How many of us need closer communion with Nature and that therapeutic environment? How many of us are lacking for a creative hobby or benevolent obsession? How many of us watch too much damn television?

Produce from your organic garden will be superior to that grown on huge corporate farms, often imported from countries where pesticide controls are different. Yours will be beautifully fresh instead of having ripened in transit. Yes, a small portion of your produce will have bug bites on it but at least the bugs will have fresh breath. Remember how much you hate to wash wax off of store-bought vegetables?

A word of caution to the novice: Take your endeavors seriously and follow through with what you've begun. I have seen people go into organic gardening with such enthusiasm and then let simple neglect rob them of harvest. Your backyard garden need not require more than an hour a day three to four days a week – ten hours a week maximum. If you want to want to grow thirty or more different kinds of food and harvest everyday it's going to require more a bit more input.

Amazingly many people don't know that homegrown, organic fruits and vegetables don't taste like the vegetables we are accustomed to from the local grocery. Much of the produce we obtain from grocery chains is grown far distant from where it is consumed. Therefore the shipper must harvest the food before ripe, often preserve it with some sort of chemicals (or worse yet, fumigate it with nuclear radiation), ship it for weeks and wax it down so that it looks appealing on display.

Quite simply, your family deserves better than this. Who will solve the problem for you? Certainly yourself.

C'mon get motivated! Visit a nursery, organic garden or library this week. You deserve a healthy prosperous life.

I highly recommend you consult gardening resources, books, nurseries and magazines, for information on inter-planting, growth rates, seasonal crops and information on virtually all types of plants that your area's climate will sustain. The books contain valuable information dealing with pests, which strains resist insects, fungi, bacteria and most any problem you will encounter. Be careful, certain books might only deal briefly with organic gardening.

Organic gardening is fun, easy, economical and a year round pursuit in climates such as my own in Southern

California.   Your family's health will reflect enhanced immune response meaning fewer colds, flu episodes, rashes, allergies, etc.   The money you will save at the grocery store will be hundreds, even thousands of dollars per year and you will be eating the freshest and finest vegetables available.

My intent is not so much to sound like an expert but to motivate as many as possible to make this self-empowering move for themselves.   As your experience grows you will develop many useful techniques for your own garden as well as discovering valuable resources for further information.   It's a winning combination for yourself and your family.   More bang for your buck, better health, a source of pride and self esteem, good exercise and a strategy for survival in this expensive and pollution filled environment.

References for An Organic Gardening Reality

Compiled largely from the NATIONAL ORGANIC DIRECTORY published by the Community Alliance with Family Farmers. (See listing under "Books")

Organizations

- California Certified Organic Farmers (CCOF) / State Office – 1115 Mission Street, Santa Cruz, CA 95060, (408)423-4528. CCOF is a membership organization of over 650 California organic growers and food processors along with an extensive support network of business and organizations.   CCOF is the primary certification and trade association of organic producers in the state and also supports research and advocacy for organic standards. Publishes a quarterly newsletter in addition to the Certified Organic Membership Directory and other consumer brochures.

- African Network on Development of Ecological Agriculture (ANDEA) – PO Box 16785, Accra-North, Ghana, Fax 233-21-228668. Contact Godsway MacBright, Program coordinator. ANDEA promotes organic farming, cottage industry and environmental protection and is made up of agriculturists, farmers and politicians.

- Midwest Organic Alliance – 5217 Wayzata Blvd. # 208, St. Louis Park, MN 55416, (612)593-2797. Contact Angela Sterns, Marketing Manager. The Alliance is non-profit and works with organic growers and processors in Minnesota, Wisconsin, Iowa, No. Dakota and So. Dakota to increase the supply of organic products. E-mail <moa7@aol.com>.

- National Coalition Against the Misuse of Pesticides (NCAMP) – 701 E Street SE, # 200, Washington, DC, (202)543-4791. Contact Sarah Sullivan. NCAMP serves as a national network committed to pesticide safety and adoption of alternative pest management techniques. Provides useful information on pesticides and publishes a quarterly magazine Pesticides and You as well as a monthly news bulletin NCAMP's Technical Report.

- National Cooperative Business Association (NCBA) – 1401 New York Ave. NW, Washington, DC, (202)638-6222, Fax 638-1374. NCBA is a national trade association and represents cooperative business. NCBA links people and organizations that share an interest in cooperative development. Publishes numerous publications for cooperative developers.

- Nature Farming Research and Development Foundation (NFRDF) – 6495 Santa Rosa Rd., Lompoc, CA 93436, (805)736-9599. Contact Susan Randall, Information Coordinator. NFRDF is dedicated to advancing natural agriculture and farming methods developed by Mokichi Okada. Operates a 75 acre Naturfarm in Lompoc which is certified organic, whose products are marketed through various outlets. Provides papers, conferences and videos as well as tours and speakers.

- Organic Growers & Buyers Association (OGBA) – 7362 University Ave., #208, Fridley, MN 55432, (612)572-1967. Contact Roni M. Brunner, Executive Director. OGBA is a third-party organic certification agency and provides services to producers, processors, manufacturers, traders and brokers worldwide. Arranges agreements with other certifiers enabling worldwide trade agreements to maintain integrity.

- NutriClean Organic Certification Program – 1 Kaiser Plaza, # 901, Oakland, CA 94612, (510)832-0359. Contact Eric Engbeck, Director. NutriClean offers domestic and international services to producers, processors, manufacturers and handlers. Requires laboratory product testing and labels to show "No Detected Residue."

Books

- The National Organic Directory – published by the Community Alliance with Family Farmers, Davis California, (800)852-3832.   Lists organic farmers, wholesalers and business by region and includes a marketing guide and index of more than 1,000 organic commodities. $35.00 plus postage.   400 pages. Perhaps the best directory for obtaining information on every aspect of sustainable agriculture, organic production and global marketing.

- Natural Resource Directory – published by Natural Resources, Inc., 520 Washington Blvd., Suite 509, Marina del Rey, CA 90292, (310)305-8521. A broad directory of health, fitness, natural remedies, natural food markets, restaurants and much more. Free to the public. "The Healthy Yellow Pages"

- Rodale's All-New Encyclopedia of Organic Gardening – published by Rodale Press, 33 East Minor Street, Emmaus, PA 18098.   A complete, practical and authoritative guide on every aspect of organic gardening. $17.95 / 690 pages.

- Step By Step Organic Vegetable Gardening – by Shepherd Ogden and published by HarperCollins Publishers Inc., 10 East 53rd Street, New York, NY 10022. The gardening classic, revised and updated in 1992. $25.00 / 299 pages.

- Taylor's Guide to Vegetables & Herbs – published by Houghton Mifflin Company, 2 Park Street, Boston MA 02108. A comprehensive pictorial encyclopedia of 198 vegetables and herbs. $16.95 / 479 pages.

- Sunset Western Garden Book – published by Lane Publishing Co., Menlo Park, CA (415)321-3600. The authority on Western Gardening for over 50 years with over 50,000 plant facts on more than 6,000 plants keyed to 24 Western climate zones. About $15.00 / 592 pages.

Magazines

- Vegetarian Times – published by Cowles Media Company. Contact info: PO Box 570, Oak Park, Il 60303, (708)848-8100. Subscription $19.97 for 8 monthly issues.

- Organic Gardening – published by Rodale Press, PO Box 7304, Red Oak, IA 51591-2304, (610)967-5171. Subscription is $25.00 per year (6 monthly and 3 bi-monthly)

- Country Living's Healthy Living – published by the Hearst Corporation, New York, NY. Contact info: PO Box 10557, Des Moines, IA 50340, (800)925-0485. As this magazine is new, subscription information has not yet been indicated. Extra copies of the premier issue (Summer 1996) are $4.95 postpaid.

- Acres U.S.A. – available from PO Box 8800, Metairie, LA 70011, (800)355-5313. Subscription is $20.00 for 12 monthly issues. Cutting edge research on eco-farming technologies, markets, analysis and trends, and extensive resources from books to herbal medicines.

- Farmer To Farmer – available from PO Box 73674, Davis, CA 95617, (916)756-7428. Subscription rate is $15.00 per year. This journal is from organic agricultural professionals and advocates for biological systems management. Avowed enemies of the agricultural chemical industry! E-mail them at <f2f@igc.apc.org>.

Index